# Raising Happy, Healthy, Safe Kids

## 50 Tips for Tackling Even the Toughest Challenges with Love, Joy, and Purpose

# Reviewing Raising Happy, Healthy, Safe Kids

This newly published book is an excellent resource for today's parents. I also recommend it for every pediatric healthcare provider and student!

The book is not a template, but a toolkit that readers can tap into. It offers concise, practical, and accessible suggestions and activities focused on providing safe, healthy environments for children to grow up in. Contemporary concepts and terminology, including gender identity, racism, bullying, and trauma-informed care, are woven throughout.

The authors acknowledge upfront that children are complicated and so are families and so is the world we live in. Yet somehow, they offer up a series of tips that are straightforward, manageable, and simple to put in place. They begin with tips on strengthening parenting and family skills, emphasizing the immediate and long-term positive role and impact they have on building resilience in children, even those in the most difficult of circumstances. Each tip helps to create a sense of safety and security, establishing a foundation and scaffolding not only for children to grow and develop, but also for them to feel confident.

No matter what your level of expertise, you will walk away with new insights and new tools for making this world a happy, healthy, and safe place for children. It doesn't get any better than that.

Martha Driessnack, PhD, PNP, RN
Emerita Faculty
OHSU School of Nursing

# Raising Happy, Healthy, Safe Kids

## 50 Tips for Tackling Even the Toughest Challenges with Love, Joy, and Purpose

**KAREN LUNDERGAN FRIESEN,** *author*

**CATHERINE E. BURNS,** *PhD, FAAN, editor*

**For
Children's Center**

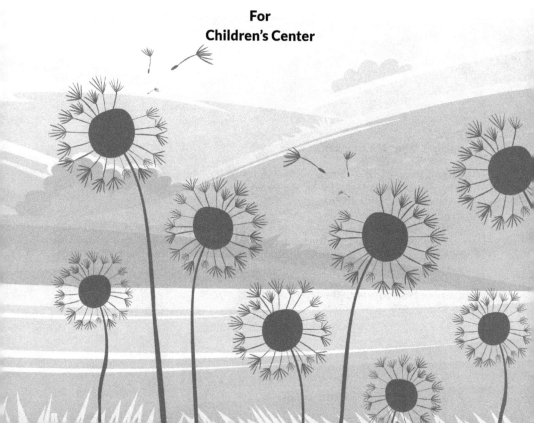

This book is dedicated to all the families, communities, and professionals who work to provide safe, healthy environments for children to grow up in, free from physical and emotional harm.

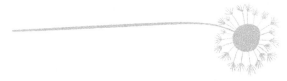

Profits from this book benefit child abuse and neglect assessment, treatment, and prevention services at

Children's Center
1710 Penn Lane,
Oregon City, OR 97045, USA

Childhelp National Child Abuse Hotline

# 1-800–4-A-CHILD
# (800)422-4453

All calls are confidential. If you need help or have questions about child abuse, call the Childhelp National Child Abuse Hotline.

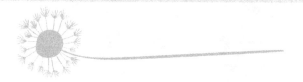

### The Dandelion
At Children's Center, the dandelion symbolizes perseverance, endurance, resilience, innocence, playfulness, and hope.
It can even grow between a rock and a hard place.
So too, children and their families can grow and thrive.

# TABLE OF CONTENTS

# INTRODUCTION

Parenting will bring you the most joy you will ever experience, and it will likely be the most difficult job you will ever have. Children are complicated! So are families, and so is the world we live in. Even if you have an "easy" child, a stable, functioning family and live in a wonderful community, your day-to-day life surely has ups and downs. So how can you emphasize the positive and minimize the problems? That's the question we asked ourselves.

Reducing the risks of child abuse and neglect is the ultimate goal of this book. Many studies have shown that when parents are in tune with their children's needs, when they have information about the risks their children face, when family members communicate well and support one another and when communities provide strong support systems to hold families up rather than pull them down, children are happier, healthier, and safer. The tips in this book provide ideas to help you strengthen your parenting skills, meet your own needs, and find support within your community to help make raising a family fun and rewarding!

## RAISING KIDS IS NOT EASY!

Children are complicated. They start out as tiny, dependent infants. Then they learn to walk and say "No!" When they enter school, they learn a whole new set of behaviors and must meet new expectations – most of which are out of your control. As teens, they take steps toward independence but don't yet have the experience and wisdom to protect themselves. The reality is, you'll never quite have the parenting role mastered because children keep changing. And each child has his or her own personality and temperament,

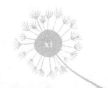

so what works for one may not work for the next. The trick is to find the joy in each stage and take pride when you figure out how to deal with the next challenge, not feel defeated when what you have been doing no longer works. It just means your child is developing at the next level. You need to develop your parenting also, just to keep up.

Families are also complicated. Two parents, teen parents, grandparents, adoptive parents, same-sex parents, single parents, step-parents and foster parents all create families and each face their unique challenges. Further, family members have different values, personalities, and interests. Some family members may come from different cultural backgrounds which influence their views about what parenting and families should be. Communication among family members may be clear or convoluted, supportive or divisive. Families also develop and change over time. Your job is to find the strengths in your family, the things that help you and support your parenting.

We are more aware of the safety threats in our world these days. Partly, this is a result of our willingness to openly consider such topics as abuse and neglect – once taboo subjects. But social media, the polarization of world views, the increasing disparities between the haves and the have-nots and many other factors outside the immediate control of you and your family impact the ways you parent and the risks your children face. It isn't all bad, though. Some families feel safer now that previously stigmatizing topics are now discussed. Tapping into your community and media resources can bolster your parenting skills in wonderful ways.

Finally, daily living is complex. Most families consist of parents who work and must also meet the needs of their children on a 24-hour basis. There's child care to think about, meals, getting the kids to soccer practice or appointments. What do you do if you or the kids are sick? How do you pay the bills? How do you get a bit of respite? It's hard to parent when you are burdened with multiple stressors.

## WHERE DID WE GET OUR INFORMATION?

In writing this book, we used information from the US Centers for Disease Control's National Center for Injury Prevention and Control, which has an entire division dedicated to violence prevention. They list 10 Family Protective Factors identified through many studies of children and families which help reduce child abuse and neglect risks for children[*]. This book offers tips and inspiration to promote the first four of these factors, all of which can be achieved at the family level. They include:

- **Nurturing parenting skills**. We can all use ideas to enhance our parenting skills.
- **Stable family relationships**. Building a stable family helps everyone – parents and kids.
- **Household rules and child monitoring**. We call this safety. Parents need to watch out for social threats to children and know what to do when problems emerge.
- **Supportive family environments and social networks**. Families do best when there is a community of support around them.

The remaining six factors – concrete support for basic needs, parental employment, parental education, adequate housing, access to health care and social services, and caring adults outside the family who can serve as role models or mentors – are beyond the scope of this book.

We also asked child development and child abuse experts to share their own personal parenting experiences as well as their knowledge about parenting practices supportive of children. Some of their personal advice and experiences are contained in the quotes at the beginning of each chapter. Also, we found current information from many national organizations and experts

---

[*] Centers for Disease Control, National Center for Injury Prevention and Control, Division of Violence Prevention, *Essentials for Childhood: Creating Safe, Nurturing Relationships and Environments for All Children, 2019.*

that provide services to children and families. We have included that resource information at the end of each tip and hope you will access all those wonderful ideas.

## HOW TO USE THIS BOOK

Think of this guide as a menu of various parenting tips which may be helpful to you as you build your parenting skills and family resources. We hope you will make the suggestions your own, adapting as you go. We added check boxes to help you consider possibilities as you read various actions, along with room for notes at the end of each tip for you to jot down your thoughts, plans, and results. What are you already doing and what can you add to your set of parenting skills?

We have also provided links to websites in order to augment our suggestions with more in-depth discussions and give you reputable places to seek help. These web-based resources are one of the most important parts of this book. Not only can they provide access to help beyond what we are able to provide, but you will quickly see that you are not the only one facing the issue at hand. You will find there are many people and organizations who have already been there and thought about the same issue you face.

We hope you will keep this book as a go-to reference you can consult as needed for guidance. Not all topics will be relevant on any given day, but over time, you will probably encounter many situations like the ones described.

We know this book cannot address all your parenting needs. Rather, consider it a toolkit with some ideas to make everyday parenting easier. It is not designed to be a template for how to parent; no one can tell you how to do that. Neither is it a good resource if a child in your home is being harmed or is at risk for harm. It is designed for prevention. Finally, it is not a resource for caring for children with significant behavioral issues. Seek help! If you or someone you know has concerns about child abuse, the Childhelp National Child Abuse Hotline (1-800-4-A-Child or 1-800-422-4453) is there for you, 24 hours a day. Our hope is this book will help you build a strong family and decrease the risks for child abuse. And we think you will find ideas that are just plain fun for your family.

## WHO CAN BENEFIT FROM THIS INFORMATION?

All caregivers—parents, grandparents, teachers, coaches, religious leaders, relatives, and friends—are essential to building safe and nurturing environments. Strong communities need *every* adult to assume responsibility not only for the well-being of their own children, but for the safety and security of every child with whom they come in contact. Ready to get started? Here are 50 ways to help you build YOUR stronger family.

# PART ONE

## BUILDING SKILLS FOR
## *Strong Nurturing*

The extent to which children's physical, emotional, and developmental needs are sensitively and consistently met.*

    Kids most definitely do not come with handbooks, but wouldn't that be nice? And, although it may *seem* as if becoming a parent should magically infuse us with endless patience and nurturing ability, those skills can take time to develop. On top of that, kids are constantly growing and evolving. As children mature, parents must also alter the strategies and skills they use to meet their kids' changing needs. Even within one family, every kid's needs are different so what works for one child may not be the best strategy for another.

---

\* Centers for Disease Control, National Center for Injury Prevention and Control, Division of Violence Prevention, *Essentials for Childhood: Creating Safe, Nurturing Relationships and Environments for All Children, 2019.*

This section provides tips to help parents or caregivers build an ever-stronger relationship with their child, with particular focus on communication and attention to emotional issues.

# 1

# SHOWER THEM *With Love*

"I love to snuggle with a newborn baby, hugging them close with their head close to mine so I can feel the warm fuzz of hair on my cheek. Hugging and kissing babies is the most natural thing in the world, and we all need hugs and kisses throughout our lives. But skillful parenting as your child grows requires being thoughtful about when, where, how much, in what way? What are the cues you need to look at to see if a hug and a kiss are right for the moment? Do you remember being a kid and not wanting to kiss your mom in front of school on the first day? What works for babies doesn't necessarily work for pre-schoolers and older, but luckily there at lots of ways to show your love."

Way back in 1976, legendary singer James Taylor introduced a famous song with a catchy chorus that goes like this:

*Shower the people you love with love*
*Show them the way you feel*
*Things are gonna be much better if you only will.*

Maybe you remember. Maybe you weren't born yet. But it's a song that continues to not only inspire enthusiastic participation in karaoke contests, but to remind us that we need to *show our love for each other.*

As it turns out, there's good reason to shower the people you love with love. It's healthy! Affection is GOOD. It's good for you. It's good for me. And it's particularly good for the kids we care about most.

Skin-to-skin contact is especially critical for newborns who rely on touch and smell to bond with parents, siblings, and other important folks in their lives. Expressions of love and connection release the "feel good" hormone oxytocin in children's brains. In addition to building trust and facilitating bonding, it launches a chemical reaction that helps kids feel good all over.

And here's what gentle, nurturing signs of love from caregivers can lead to as kids grow up:

- Greater success in school (physical touch actually stimulates brain growth)
- Physical growth (along with the oxytocin boost, growth hormones are activated)
- Fewer – or at least shorter – tantrums
- Less stress (hugging reduces stress hormones, which can lead to a lifetime of positive effects)
- Better health (here's oxytocin again, pulling double duty)
- Increased self-esteem
- Happier adults

As kids get older, they will naturally begin to shy away from cuddling, and physical affection needs to occur with their consent. That's okay. It's important to respect each child's personality-driven preferences for displays of affection, and to touch them in ways that make them feel comfortable and secure – not awkward or ashamed.

Ask them: "Want a hug?" "Kisses for you?" By age three, they can tell you if they want a hug or not – and you can still find ways to show your affection. Teaching kids to choose whether they want a hug helps them get in touch with their feelings and strengthens them on their journey of deciding to be affectionate or not with other people. By the time they become teens, children should be able to say "no" to unwanted affectionate acts in lots of situations.

Children need a safe place, physically close to their real-life heroes, when they feel scared or nervous. When caregivers look them in the eye, give them attention, smile at them and show physical and verbal affection, they will feel loved, valued, and safe. Your job is to be there when those stressful times occur and to give your affection at the time it is needed. Sometimes just a soft touch on the shoulder is enough. Bottom line: kids *need* affection. So, show them unconditional love. It's the best kind there is.

## HUG IT OUT.

Parents, there are plenty of healthy, bond-building ways to share affection with your kids.

Try this:

- ☐ **Hold, touch, and rock your baby.** Infant massage works too.

- ☐ **When holding your child's hand, teach them that three gentle squeezes represent "I love you."** It's a sweet, private message you can share anytime, anywhere.

- ☐ **Offer regular, gentle pats on the back 'just because.'** Make these gestures a part of your daily routine. Physical connections multiple times a day are important.

- ☐ **Say "I love you" every day.**

- ☐ **Give hugs or show other gentle forms of touch, even while disciplining.** This helps communicate the message that "I didn't love what you did, but I love you."

- ☐ **Ask "Want a hug?"** then let them decide.

## AMPLIFY YOUR EFFORTS.

- ☐ Write your child a sweet letter, or slip a note of encouragement into their lunchbox.

- ☐ Share favorite memories of your children with them on a regular basis.

- ☐ Look for opportunities to compliment your kids.

- ☐ Hold hands and snuggle together after asking if they want this affection.

- ☐ Talk to your child about making choices about when they need close touch such as hugs and kisses and when they are okay to deal with stresses without hugs of support.

If you're not already doing it, start showering the children *you* love with love. But don't assume that a hug and kiss every time is the right thing. Let them tell you what they want. They'll certainly benefit from it. And so will you.

## RESOURCES:

Ardiel EL, Rankin CH: *The importance of touch in development.* Available at: www.ncbi.nlm.nih. gov/pmc/articles/PMC2865952/.

Darkness to Light: *Healthy touch for children and youth.* Stewards of Children. Available at: https://www.d2l.org/education/additional-training/healthy-touch-children/

Mayo Clinic Staff: *Infant massage: understand this soothing therapy,* 2020. Available at: www.mayoclinic.org/healthy-lifestyle/infant-and-toddler-health/in-depth/infamassage/art-20047151.

Parenting for Brain: *Hugging – 7 benefits for you and your child (backed by science).* Available at: www. parentingforbrain.com/children-hugging/.

Schwartz S: *How a parent's affection shapes a child's happiness for life.* Available at: www.parent.com/how-a-parents-affection-shapes-a-childs-happiness-for-life/.

You Are Mom: *Children have a right to not kiss if they don't want to.* 2018. Available at: https://youaremom.com/children-have-a-right-not-to-kiss-if-they-dont-want-to/

---

# NOTES:

# 2

## LISTEN

"When my daughter was born it only took a few times hearing her 'hungry cry' to learn what distinguished it from 'tired cry' or 'uncomfortable cry.' Most importantly, we quickly learned all of the other cues that came before crying – wiggling, facial expressions, yawning. It felt like we'd cracked this amazing code when we were able to accurately guess which need was being communicated without waiting for crying. However, as she became a toddler and started behaviors like tantrums and 'NO', we instead began to think of her actions as problems that needed to be managed rather than the logical (to her) way to get her needs met. We had to learn that her actions weren't problems, just new ways of communicating. We needed new listening skills to anticipate her needs when possible, offer understanding of her feelings being big and real for her, and respond in a way that built trust and connection rather than isolation."

Shhhh. Do you hear that? Your child is trying to tell you something. Whether it's a happily gurgling newborn, a screaming toddler, a chatty tween or steely teenage silence, your kids are communicating.

As humans we are constantly communicating about our experiences – through words, body language and actions. Children, in particular, tend to gravitate toward the latter two as a way to clue

8

us in to what they're feeling. It can be challenging, and hard to accurately translate. But as adults, it is a wonderful gift to the children we care for to practice child-specific listening.

From the moment a newborn baby is placed in our arms, we are on a mission to figure out who they are and what they need. Typically, we become adept at hearing what they are 'saying', even when our children have no concept of language. It takes effort to learn the language of a young child or toddler, but just as with that newborn, accurately listening to your kids and helping them feel understood builds trust and attachment. It also leads them to develop greater emotional regulation.

As your children grow, their needs become more complicated – navigating school and peer relationships, gaining more responsibility, mastering difficult skills – and their methods of communication become more sophisticated to match. You may soon find you're no longer trying to discern that newborn wail, but that you're also at a loss as to what your kid is really trying to tell you in words.

Listening for the meaning behind the words (or actions) is a skill. Your investment in learning that mysterious language is a solid step toward sealing a strong parent-child bond.

## SHARPEN YOUR FREQUENCY.

You can help set the stage for high-quality communication in a few ways.

☐ **Get down to your child's eye level** (we're talking little ones here, not your six-foot teen). Set aside distractions like your laptop or phone. Then, take a critical look at your surroundings – and your own actions – from a child's point of view. Are you in a hurry? Feeling tired? Distracted by other issues? Push yourself to get in their zone.

☐ **Think "open."** Say "Tell me about that" or "What do you think about that?" "Wow...I see...Really?" Using open posture and body language expresses that you are paying attention and ready to hear.

☐ **Keep open lines of communication throughout your daily activities.** Specific check-in times are great – such as at bedtime, family dinner, or school pick-up, but don't limit your availability to listen only to set times. Your child's best time may be different from yours.

☐ **Reflect what you think is being communicated by restating and repeat it back for your child.** Clarify with "Do you mean...?" or summarize what you heard and ask "Did I get that right?" It's also okay to do some guessing and provide a name for feelings that your child may not otherwise have the capacity to express. This helps show your understanding and teaches kids emotional literacy.

☐ **Empathetic listening is important.** Affirm your child's feelings by saying "I can see how angry you are" or "Tell me more...how are you feeling?" Focusing on the behavior alone can be a missed opportunity. Watch your child's body language to see what else they are communicating.

☐ **Pay attention to their behavior and physical cues.** Not all listening relies on words, especially with children. Body aches and physical complaints can often clue you in to a child's emotional needs. For example, a stomachache might actually be communicating anxiety or fear. A child acting out or misbehaving is trying to communicate a need, but may not have the language ability or insight to ask directly. Go ahead and ask for clarification. "Is someone hurting you?" or "Are you afraid to go to school?"

## AMPLIFY YOUR EFFORTS.

As for that six-foot teenager hunkered down in the bedroom upstairs? Here's a not-so-secret secret: he can talk, but he still might be a poor communicator. Changes in your kids' communication style is a natural part of growing up, and listening at this stage of your child's life may be more important than ever before. Here's how you can step up your game:

- ☐ **Suppress your default "parent response" urge when your teen comes to you with a need or concern.** Don't judge. Don't overreact.

- ☐ **Stay calm, regardless of what your gut may be doing.**

- ☐ **Remember, you are a sounding board.** To the best of your ability, keep your responses neutral on topics of great emotion. Your kids need you to be their supporter and their 'rock.'

- ☐ **Expect your child to speak appropriately.** You are not obligated to listen to insults, yelling, threats, etc.

- ☐ **Recognize that devoting your full attention sends the critical message to your teen that they are worth listening to.** That investment will build trust and encourage more open communication.

---

# RESOURCES:

Centers for Disease Control and Prevention: *Essentials for Parenting Toddlers and Preschoolers. Active Listening.* November, 2019. Available at: https://www.cdc.gov/paarents/essentials/communication/activelistening.html (Also in Spanish)

National Center on the Sexual Behavior of Youth. Available at: https://ncsby.org/content/communicating- your-adolescent

Newman C: *5 Easy ways to be a better listener to your child,* September 11, 2020. Available at: www.parents.com/parenting/better-parenting/advice/easy-ways-to-be-a-better-listener-to-your-child/

# NOTES:

# 3
# *Read* OUT LOUD

"As both a clinician and mom with two young children, I'm fascinated by how much I learn about children's internal experiences when we read together. As they explore the thoughts and feelings of different characters in books, I get to hear how they think and feel about what goes on in the world. Many of the best discussions I've had with both my own children and clients began by reading a book!"

Let's reflect for a moment on the old adage that goes something like "A book a day keeps the badness away." Not ringing any bells? Okay, so it's not an actual saying, but maybe it *should* be. Why? Because reading to children is good for their brains, and it's great for building lasting bonds and memories.

Among its widely-recognized benefits, reading aloud to children:

- Develops language, speech, and communication skills
- Improves concentration
- Promotes logical thinking
- Builds imagination
- Instills empathy
- Introduces new vocabulary, ideas, experiences, people, and places

All that, from a few words on a page. Best of all, reading aloud with children is fun— filled with protagonists and antagonists, mystery and adventure, talking animals and wacky characters.

Television, text messages, e-mail and other pursuits pull parents in different directions. But by putting aside these diversions to read with your children—even for just a few minutes a day—you show them your love. Bedtime reading can be especially gratifying. And the time you invest now will pay significant dividends later.

## CHECK IT OUT.

The beauty of this adult-child bonding phenomenon is in its simplicity: grab a book, sit down together, and go. Within moments, you'll be meeting new people, traveling to new places and off on exciting adventures – all while building intellectual potential in the little people you care about most.

☐ **Reading together any time of the day is encouraged**—but try to carve out at least one designated reading time that kids can count on. Reading at bedtime is a great way to wind down each day—and it's a ritual kids love. Encourage comments and conversation as you read, and keep it lively!

☐ **Reading requires that all electronics be turned off**. That's harder for older kids to do. Try to make it a routine of the evening – turn off the cell phone, read, then turn out the light.

☐ **Offer a variety of stories.** While there are benefits to reading children the same stories over and over (it contributes to developing that logical thinking ability), reciting "Goodnight Moon" six times a day for 19 consecutive weeks can be mind-numbing for the average adult. So, stock up! Public libraries are treasure troves. They're free! Thrift stores and garage sales are also great places for finding new stories.

Looking for some fresh material? Ask your local children's

librarian for suggestions, swap books with friends, and don't forget some of these:

- *Where the Wild Things Are*
- *The Very Hungry Caterpillar*
- *Last Stop on Market Street*
- *The Snowy Day*
- *Lola at the Library*
- *Alexander and the Terrible, Horrible, No Good, Very Bad Day*
- *The Giving Tree*
- *Guess How Much I Love You*
- *Amelia Bedelia*
- *Charlotte's Web*
- *Mango, Abuela, and Me*
- *Danbi Leads the School Parade*
- *At the Mountain's Base*
- *Return to Sender*
- *How It All Blew Up*
- *The King of Kindergarten*
- *Stand Up, Yumi Chang*

As your kids grow, keep up the tradition. Experts say that reading together even into the teenage years remains beneficial. Choose books that will challenge your teen, introduce new topics, and inspire dialogue.

## AMPLIFY YOUR EFFORTS.

☐ **You don't have to be a parent to read to a kid.** Most schools have programs that welcome volunteers as readers and tutors. Type "helping children read" and your town's name into any search engine to locate other local opportunities.

☐ **Check out resources at the local library.** Most public libraries host regular read-aloud programs for toddlers and young children. Often, music and other educational activities are included. Listening to recorded books is another great way to pass the time during car rides and doesn't require an adult to read directly. Books about other cultures help kids learn about diversity.

For families who read in languages other than English: Enjoy reading in your primary language. What a gift for your child to be able to read and speak multiple languages!

☐ **Donate books or financial gifts to a reading-focused organization**. A little contribution can make a huge impact. The Ferst Foundation for Childhood Literacy (www.ferst-foundation.org) mails new books to thousands of children each month—one per month through their fifth birthday, at no charge to eligible families. Focused on children from low-income communities in Georgia, and funded largely by donations, this creative initiative costs just $36 per child annually. And for a few more dollars, "gift subscriptions" are available to families *anywhere*.

The bottom line: by reading aloud to a child, or by making it easier for others to do so, you *will* be helping to change a life. In the process, you may be helping to change the world.

---

# RESOURCES:

African-American Literary Book Club: *Top 12 recommended African-American children's books*. Available at: http://www.aalbc.com/books/children

Anti-defamation League: *9 Must-read children's books for National Hispanic Heritage Month*, 2021. Available at: www.adl.org/blog/9-must-read-childrens-books-for-national-hispanic-heritage-month.

Giorgis C: *Jim Trelease's Read Aloud Handbook* 8th ed. 2019, New York Public Library: *100 Great children's books/100 years*. Available at: www.nypl.org/childrens100.

Oklahoma's Glenpool Fire Department Dads: *The brainy benefits of bedtime stories*. Available at: www.parents.com/fun/entertainment/books/the-brainy-benefits-of-bedtime-stories/.

One Tough Job. org: 1000 books before kindergarten – one tough job. Available at: www.onetoughjob.org/articles/1000-books-before-kindergarten/

Reading Rockets. Available at: www.readingrockets.org/. (Website).

Parents Editors. 26 best books for Latino Kids. 2022. Available at: https://www.parents.com/fun/entertainment/books/20-best-books-for-latino-kids/

PBSSoCal: *12 Children's books to celebrate Asian-American Pacific Island Heritage Month*, 2021. Available at: www.pbssocal.org/education/famiies/12-books-to-celebrate-asian-american-paific-island-heritage-month

# NOTES:

# 4

## HELP GUIDE THEIR *Feelings*

"I had a nighttime routine when my kids were younger where, after their story as they were being tucked into bed, they spent a few minutes talking about their day. I would ask them what was the best thing that happened that day, what was the worst thing that happened and then I asked them what they felt and why. I was able to amplify the good things and talk about how the worst thing could have been made better. Sometimes I'd share what my best and worst moments were. Reflecting on feelings in a quiet moment is a wonderful time for sharing and helping kids get in touch with their emotions, and it works with preschoolers well into school age."

Remember that epic tantrum your little one had at Target? As if you could ever forget. Kids' emotions can seem so...BIG. Anger, sadness, joy, fear, frustration. When young children experience these feelings, they let us know it – often with exuberance and volume. Part of a child's job is learning how to communicate and manage their emotions – both the highs and lows. Like any new skill, figuring it all out takes practice and guidance.

Feelings are neither right nor wrong. They simply are. But there can be more or less healthy ways to express them. Bottling up emotions over the long haul is as unproductive as a Target tantrum

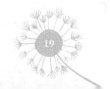

and, experts say, can actually shorten a person's life by making them more susceptible to stress-related diseases.

Managing life's roller coaster of emotions is a forever sort of project. But as parents and supporters of growing children, here's what's important to know right now: 1) It's actually okay for small children to throw down the occasional, awful tantrum. It's part of the process and proves they are not, in fact, robots. 2) You get to help them grow through this stage, teaching coping skills for expressing and managing all their feelings – good and bad.

We owe it to our kids and to the people who come into their orbit to teach them "feelings management" that is healthy, balanced and fitting for the circumstances.

## LET IT OUT.

Ground rule number one: Be a positive role model. Because guess who's listening from the backseat when you get fed up in traffic and unleash a verbal tirade? Kids are always listening and looking to you to learn how to manage situations that come with big feelings.

Some of the ways that you can have a positive impact:

☐ **Show kids that you have feelings too.** Making statements like "I know you are sad that you didn't get to go to your friend's house today. Sometimes I am sad when I can't do what I want to do, too," or "I'm so tired. I think I should get to bed early" indicates you "get it," you recognize negative or challenging feelings within yourself, and you have a plan for how to deal with them. And remember to let out a whoop when something good happens too!

☐ **Look for the reasons behind moods and behavior.** Did they miss a nap? Are they struggling in school or over-scheduled? Are they toddlers simply trying to communicate? Is someone hurting them – through bullying or other abusive behaviors? Regardless of age, *understanding* behavior and being aware of what causes your child stress can help you select the right approach.

☐ **Name that feeling**. Teach kids about emotions. Learning words that describe emotions can help your child identify them and then communicate with you. So, talk about being angry, happy, sad, embarrassed and so on as a normal part of your day. Say things like: "It's so exciting that you scored a goal!" "I know you feel frustrated that we have to leave the park, but we'll come back another day." Or, "Yes, sometimes it is scary when the lights are out. But you're safe in your bed." You can also talk about characters in books and on TV also, asking "How do you think he is feeling right now?"

☐ **Recommend ways to tackle strong feelings.** Perhaps it's reading a book or running around in the yard. Sometimes hanging out in their special place in the home is the ticket. Drawing, dance, writing, and music are all helpful ways to manage feelings. The goal here is to teach kids about the resources that exist within and around them to help build coping skills and to learn to separate feelings from behaviors.

Taking deep breaths, counting, taking a break, problem-solving, and identifying mood boosters like reading a book or going for a walk are all excellent ways to help kids calm down and cope with their feelings. Be sure to reward their efforts!

☐ **Let them cry.** It's like a giant emotional release valve. Also, avoid making a big deal out of big emotions. If you remain calm, there's a good chance your worked-up child will soon be able to dial it down as well. Aim to be caring and responsive. It's important for children to know you're there to support them.

☐ **Teach and model empathy** – and awareness of the feelings of others.

## AMPLIFY YOUR EFFORTS.

Teenagers require special care and handling in the feelings department. It's typical for some of them to become more distant and non-communicative during these years. Trying to figure out what's bothering them without being an interrogator can feel impossible.

Your challenge? To support teens in navigating their emotions without being overly nosy or intrusive (again, not an easy road). Try these tactics:

☐ **Allow your teen time and space to process what's going on – maybe alone in their favorite space, on a walk, talking with friends or engaging in other positive activities.**

☐ **Reassure them that their feelings are legitimate, and that they can talk with you about anything.**

☐ **Remain calm – and don't jump to conclusions or take sides. Parent freak-outs do little to calm emotional teens.**

☐ **Seek professional help from your pediatric health care provider, school counselor or a pediatric mental health expert if you are concerned about your child's emotions.**

Emotions can be big, but they shouldn't get in the way of everyday life. Sadness, anger, anxiety – these are feelings that can interfere with learning and building friendships. Teens who start to do poorly in school, start isolating, have dramatic changes in sleep patterns, develop self-destructive/risky behaviors, or have a preoccupation with death need to be carefully monitored and should receive counseling right away

Suffering from anxiety, depression, substance abuse, grief, attention deficit disorder or being bullied or abused are just a few of the factors that can lead to emotions spiraling out of control and should involve the support of a professional. If you are worried about the immediate safety of your child, call your local emergency services or **Childhelp** number right away.

And in the midst of this full-speed-ahead parenting gig, don't forget to take care of your own emotional health. For all your hard work, *your* feelings deserve some TLC, too.

---

# RESOURCES:

Ehmke R: *Helping children deal with grief.* Child Mind Institute. Available at: https://childmind.org/article/helping-children-deal-grief/ (Also in Spanish)

Gustafson T: *Keeping your emotions bottled up could kill you,* 2018. Available at: https://www.huffpost.com/archive/ca/entry/bottling-up-negative-emotions_b_5056433

Morin A: *How to help an overly emotional child cope with their feelings,* 2019. Available at: https://www.verywellfamily.com/how-to-help-an-overly-emotional-child-4157594

Orson K: *10 reasons your toddler's tantrum is actually a good thing,* 2019. Available at: www.mondaymorningmomschildcare.com/post/10-reasons-your-toddlers-tantrum-is-actually-a-good-thing

# NOTES:

# 5

# ANSWER ALL THEIR *Questions*

> "Remember how when we were kids and we'd ask our parents or teachers a question, and they'd blush and say, 'I'll tell you when you're older,' or, 'You're not ready for that yet'? It's infuriating for kids! They want to learn, and we have the obligation to figure out how to teach them about 'difficult' subjects gently, responsibly, and appropriately."

When your kid asks you an uncomfortable question (think: "How did I get inside your tummy?" "Why did Grandpa have to die?" or "Why can't we afford _____?"), what is your go-to reaction? Do you:

a) Give a "feel good answer" even though it might not be true?
b) Hand over a copy of Gray's Anatomy or Money magazine and tell them to "study up!"
c) Look your child straight in the eye and answer them succinctly and thoroughly.
d) None of the above.

Perhaps the first question here should be "why do kids ask so many questions?" Because, for real, a curious child at the peak of their question-asking career (around four years old) bombards mom and dad with close to 100 questions a day. There are simply bound to be some zingers in there. So, are we obligated to answer them all?

Apparently, yes. Meaning, at least the big ones. Of course, we want to encourage curiosity and learning as much as possible and all those questions mean we've got vibrant little sponges on our hands. It's just that some questions are much harder to tackle than others, either because they're awkward or we literally don't know the answer. But answering our kids directly and honestly ensures children know they are respected and listened to, and that you are a trusted source of information. And, thanks to Google and child-rearing professionals, you're covered. So now what?

## BE FEARLESS.

Don't be intimidated by either toddlers or teens! After all, they just want to know stuff!

☐ **When younger children ask difficult questions, be encouraging and reassuring.** Say, "Good question! Thank you for asking." Make sure they know it's always okay to come to you with whatever is on their mind. As you answer, be honest and direct. It's perfectly okay to acknowledge that something is uncomfortable, but don't avoid any topic.

☐ **Take your time, but don't ignore or avoid their questions.** When a query comes out of the blue (which is pretty much life with kids), you may need time to think – or even do a little research – to come up with an age-appropriate response. Maybe you've been hit with a "why is that man so old?" in a crowded grocery line. Don't hesitate to say: "Let's talk about that when we get back to the car/at bedtime/after school so I can give you my full attention." Then be sure you do just that.

☐ **Keep it age appropriate.** Answering questions doesn't mean you need to use graphic words or concepts, tell them all the details about how you feel about your ex, your issues around finances, or any number of other topics that don't relate directly to their lives. Try to answer their questions in a way that doesn't raise fears for them. For example, say "I'm trying to use our money so it helps us the most" rather than "We don't have enough money." Further, your answers need to be consistent with their developmental and academic level.

☐ **Listen and ask questions yourself.** Follow up with "Does that make sense?" Or "Do you have any other questions about this?" If the child wants a fuller answer, do your best to accommodate. There is a good chance they will simply say "okay" and move on to something else.

☐ **Start early.** Make difficult topics part of your routine early on and you'll find they become much less intimidating as your children grow. Going over body safety rules at a young age, for instance, is critical. Approaching it with a no-nonsense confidence will make it easier to discuss even heftier adolescent topics later on – such as pornography, social media presence, sex and relationships, and consent for intimacy. Frame your answers within the context of your own family values.

As your kids approach the teen years, they may become less communicative, but it's even more important to encourage their questions. Help create a teen-friendly atmosphere by keeping these things in mind:

☐ **Be thoughtful about where you are and who is around when broaching a subject.** Keep in mind that your child may be reluctant to discuss some subjects with their peers or other people around.

☐ **Stay open minded.** Don't jump to conclusions when your child asks something provocative.

- ☐ **Don't lecture or overshare about your own experiences.** This isn't about you.

- ☐ **Validate their feelings** – even if you don't necessarily agree with them.

- ☐ **Guide your child to problem solve and troubleshoot difficult questions or situations.**

- ☐ **Offer advice only when asked** (but it's okay to ask them if they would like your advice!)

- ☐ **Make sure they know that if they want your help, all they need to do is ask.**

## AMPLIFY YOUR EFFORTS.

Maximize those fleeting one-on-one opportunities, like car rides. While starting difficult conversations with a child or teen may initially feel awkward, you'll ultimately end up creating space for genuine emotional sharing and exploration. When conducted sincerely, both you and your child will end up feeling more connected and understood. On the other hand, don't trap kids in those car ride situations if they don't want to engage in the conversation you had in mind.

Here's another idea – start asking your kids the questions. It will get them talking. They can be really out-of-the-box ones too. See the Kids-R-Kids resource below for 63 good ones. (Magee, 2019).

And remind yourself of this hard fact: If YOU don't answer your kids' questions from an early age and talk to them about the difficult topics, they'll find someone else who will.

# RESOURCES:

Edmunds M: *10 Answers to your teen's uncomfortable questions.* How stuff works. Available at: https://health.howstuffworks.com/pregnancy-and-parenting/teenage-health/10-answers-to-teen-questions.htm

Magee E: *63 fun questions to get your kid talking*, November, 2019. Available at: https://kidsrkids.com/jersey-village/2019/11/10/63-fun-questions-to-get-your-kid-talking/

McKenna C: *How to talk to a 5-year-old about porn.* Oct. 5, 2016. Available at: https://www.protectyoungeyes.com/how-to-talk-to-a-5-year-old-about-porn/

Turner C & Kamenetz A: *When kids ask (really) tough questions: A quick guide.* Feb. 28, 2019. Available at: www.npr.org/2019/02/28/698304854/when-kids-ask-really-tough-questions-a-quick-guide.

ParentInfo: *Three tips for starting a difficult conversation with your child.* May, 2018. Available at: www.parentinfo.org/article/three-tips-for-starting-a-difficult-conversation-with-your-child.

# NOTES:

# 6

# SET CLEAR *Boundaries*

"When my children were young, my partner and I would have the best intentions for family game nights. Inevitably, something would go wrong for my preschool son—causing him to lose a turn, be sent back to start, or somehow realize he just may not end up the winner. The game board would be flipped by his little chubby hands and the plan for evening family bonding and joyous together time would turn into crying children, frustrated parents, and game pieces everywhere! How quickly we realized it was up to us to teach him to understand and deal with his emotions in an appropriate way if he was ever going to successfully navigate a future of competitive fun with others! Investing time in setting some behavioral boundaries along with teaching, modeling, practice, persistence, and praise led to many successful game nights and eventually an athlete who enjoys competition and is even known as a good sport!"

You may relate to this scenario: Kid #1 is relentlessly curious and creative, Yesterday she "decorated" your bathroom wall with crayons and today she built a "garden" in your kitchen. For the sake of family health and happiness, you need to set some boundaries, stat!

We hear this term a lot, but what does "setting boundaries" even mean? According to parenting expert Debbie Pincus, we

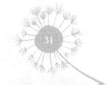

can think of a boundary as "the line you draw around yourself to define where you end and where your child begins." It also means just straight up setting some limits and rules.

How do limits help kids – and parents? In tons of ways, it turns out. Here's what solid boundaries and limits can do:

**Prepare kids for the real world.** Growing up with rules and clear boundaries sets kids up for success, equipping them with the skills they need to build positive relationships with friends, co-workers and family members.

**Create a sense of order.** When small kids know what is expected of them, they often eagerly comply. This could mean simple things, like brushing their teeth at night or not eating food on the furniture. Rules create order, and though kids are bound to attempt to wriggle around your expectations, there are plenty of ways in which they will cooperate. Just listen in when their friends come over and they quickly inform them how things are done at your place. Playing games with rules to follow is a great place to practice working within boundaries too.

**Build confidence – and competence.** Clear rules send a message to kids that they don't have to constantly test the boundaries They will try, but as they mature and demonstrate their ability to follow your family guidelines, earning new privileges provides incentive to keep it up. And with new privileges and independence comes confidence.

**Provide reassurance.** As much as any respectable teenager would beg to differ, there IS some relief in knowing that parents are in charge, and that somebody is paying attention to their choices and actions.

**Keep them safe.** It's why we make kids wear bike helmets and seatbelts and hold hands in the crosswalk and keep matches locked up. Plenty of rules exist to protect them, us, and others.

# DRAW THE LINE.

What about consequences? In order for rules and limits to get your kids' attention, there needs to be a down side to breaking them.

A few thoughts:

☐ **Make sure the discipline fits the situation.** Consequences should be appropriate and consistent with the circumstances. Grounding your teenager for six months for breaking curfew or imposing a five-hour time out for a four-year-old may sound about right in the heat of the moment, but we all know that's going too far. Decide on a logical consequence for the action, one that will teach a lesson in a firm, relevant, but ultimately loving way.

☐ **It's okay to delay the consequence,** particularly with older children. Tell your child: "I'm too upset to decide what the consequence is. I need some time to think about it, and we'll talk later." This will give you a chance to cool down and think straight, while at the same time force your child to review their behavior.

☐ **Hold firm to your rules and boundaries.** Ignoring poor behavior because you don't want to deal with an unpleasant interaction is surprisingly tempting at times, but bound to backfire. Family rules are made to be followed, and assuming yours are clear, fair, and reasonable for the child's age, it's your job to enforce them. You'll teach your kids responsibility and demonstrate that you are a parent who has enough self-respect to set the bar and stick to your word. Note: rules will need to change as kids grow up. Make sure they understand ahead of time when a new rule is established.

☐ **Be consistent.** It's confusing to children to be able to get away with something on a Tuesday only to be disciplined for the same thing on Friday. It also leads to more limit-testing as they attempt to assess where you really plan to draw the line. Prepare to be flexible, but not unreliable.

☐ **Accentuate the positive.** When their behavior is great, notice it and tell them! A heartfelt "I really appreciate the way you cleaned up your toys today" may just get you even more tomorrow. Another note on positivity: try framing rules with positive language. For example, try replacing "no backtalking," with "use kind and respectful words."

☐ **Get kids involved.** As the parent, you have the final say on boundary lines, but you might consider letting your kids weigh in. If they have a stake in outlining expectations, they may be more likely to comply. You can even ask them what they think a reasonable consequence could be for a clear infraction of the rules. On that note, avoid making a truck-load of rules. That's just exhausting for everybody. Rather, stick to a handful of clear, meaningful ones and be prepared to change and widen the boundaries as your child matures.

☐ **Try to keep consequences fair.** Siblings are always watching, and no doubt they will jump at an opportunity to point out when they feel they've been wronged. If you choose to dole out a different form of discipline for a similar infraction, be prepared to explain why. It could be: "She has never done that before. You did it three times," or "He isn't as old as you were." And a gentle reminder: keep consequences age appropriate and be sure you and any parenting partners are in sync when it comes to managing discipline.

## AMPLIFY YOUR EFFORTS.

Work to 'catch' your kids doing things the right way and point it out. Your home shouldn't become a rule-bound castle but a welcome and nurturing place to be. Emphasize the positive!

Until they approach adulthood, it's crucial to remember our children are kids – not our best friends, our peers, or our most trusted confidants. So, teach kids to knock before they walk into your bedroom. Teach them not to interrupt conversations. And, keep yourself from leaning on them in the midst of relationship problems or other stresses you are facing.

Let them be kids. That's a big enough job for now.

## RESOURCES:

All Pro Dad: *10 ways to establish clear boundaries for children*, 2018. Available at: www.allprodad. com/10-ways-to-establish-clear-boundaries-for-children/.

Neifert M: *Why kids need rules*, 2019. Available at: https://www. parenting.com/child/why-kids-need-rules/

Pincus D: *Parental roles: how to set healthy boundaries with your child*, 2021. Available at: http://www.empoweringparents.com/article/ parental-roles-how-to-set-healthy-boundaries-with-your-child/

# NOTES:

# 7
# CHOOSE YOUR *Struggles*

"Every day there's at least one opportunity for a power struggle with my three-year-old. I've learned to expect them. If I'm not careful, something small—such as who removes my son's shoes—can turn into a full-blown temper tantrum. As soon as I think something has been figured out, it changes again! It can be maddening but I've learned to 'go with the flow' for things that are a big deal to him, but not a big deal for me. Arguing about shoes is not worth my energy—or his!"

Around age two, children wake up to the fact that they are separate from their parents. Once that realization dawns, they begin exploring ways to exert their independence, a process that typically doesn't completely stop until they're independent adults. In other words, buckle in. It's gonna be a long ride!

The anatomy of a power struggle with a child boils down to four simple components:

1. You want your child to do a particular thing or behave in a particular way.
2. They don't feel like it and respond accordingly.
3. You're not about to give in. They're not about to give in.
4. Conflict ensues.

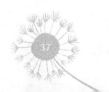

Clearly, there are no winners.

On the surface, a power struggle might *appear* to be a battle over forced vegetable eating, or cleaning up toys, or whether or not it's appropriate to wear a cape to school. But at the heart of every power struggle is control: a child's desire to gain it, and your desire to maintain it.

Even the tiniest humans need to feel like they have some control over their world. And truth is, kids need to grow that confidence in order to evolve into strong adults who know how to make solid decisions. Your job is to allow them to have some control while still keeping them safe, healthy and on track with your family values.

As it turns out, there *are* some techniques that work to defuse power struggles. By (counterintuitively) yielding some power to your child, you can also achieve your goals and effectively eliminate the "struggle" from almost any power struggle.

## DROP THE ROPE.

No, really. Stop the tug of war.

Stop, breathe and ask yourself this: Why is this happening right now? Is my child tired, hungry, or emotional for some other reason? And, what can I do to put a stop to this challenging behavior when I'm exhausted, frustrated and my child is currently testing boundaries?

First, quickly evaluate whether what you want your child to do or not do is a 'non-negotiable' issue such as wearing a seatbelt, holding hands when crossing the street, or turning off an inappropriate movie and, if it is, by all means insist that your expectations are followed.

But if the issue at hand is something you can honestly let go of, remind yourself that giving up a power struggle does not have to be the same thing as 'giving in.' Once you realize you've stepped too far into a disagreement, you can save face – and save the day – by saying something like: "Okay. We've both had a long day. Let's start over," and take it from there.

Some time-tested approaches:

☐ **Offer your child a choice.** Giving them a say places some control in their hands while also meeting your objective. "It's naptime. Do you want to walk to your room or would you like me to carry you?" Or, "Would you like to eat a bite of carrot or a bite of fruit?"

☐ **Allow for natural consequences to unfold.** Case study: mealtime. Even when you offer choices, you can't actually force a child to eat. If they choose not to, eventually they'll get hungry. It's nature's way of solving the problem. And, nope. If they don't eat the veggies, they don't get the cookie.

☐ **When a power struggle appears imminent, react calmly and consistently.** Kids will learn that their behavior has no power over you, which can cut short outbursts and cut down their frequency.

☐ **Ask them how they think you should resolve the situation.** This works best with slightly older kids – inviting them to evaluate what is unfolding, and hopefully learning to see multiple sides of an issue. But even three-year-olds can negotiate! And negotiation is a perfectly acceptable approach to resolution.

☐ **Approach the conflict as a way to hone your skills.** When you succeed at turning a situation around and stopping a power struggle in its tracks? Wow, giant fist pump.

## AMPLIFY YOUR EFFORTS.

Consider this section "Power Struggles: Teen Edition." Conflicts with adolescents probably feel a lot like the ones you experienced during the toddler years – only this time the stakes are higher and your decisions about how and where to spend your energy will be tested mightily.

Child-rearing experts recommend keeping an open mind when it comes to some things, so that you can firmly hold your ground on others. A few areas where you might allow a pass in order to keep your relationship intact? Room cleanliness, music genres, hair length, food choices, clothing (for the most part), sleep schedules. However, safety is essential. Hold firm on those issues.

Within each of these categories, of course, there are limits to acceptability – and it's your right and obligation to enforce them. But showing you are reasonable about some things sets you up for more success in making headway with your teen on the issues that matter more.

---

# RESOURCES:

Lavoie R: *Flip the switch on the power struggle*, 2021. Available at: https://additudemag.com/power-struggles-adhd-kids-teachers/

Sims K: *Dealing with power struggles*, 2015. Available at: https://gwcac.va.networkofcare.org/mh/library/article.aspx?id=2408

Tamm L: *4 Ridiculously easy ways to end a power struggle*, 2021. Available at: https://themilitarywifeandmom.com/how-to-stop-toddler-power-struggles/

# NOTES:

# 8

# *Try Saying* "YES, AND...."

"The first rule you learn in improv is to respond to an offer with 'Yes, and...' Saying 'yes' means you accept another person's creative thought. 'And' is an agreement to build upon it – helping fan the creative spark into a flame. 'Yes, and' doesn't have to be confined to the world of improv, though. I try to use 'yes, and' whenever I spend time with my nieces and nephews, and it always results in funny and memorable experiences."

SCENE 1 (the family room):

CHILD: I'm so hot I wish I could eat the world's biggest ice cream cone.

YOU: Oh, *yes. And* if you could build the world's biggest ice cream cone, I bet it would be 10 stories tall and have 152 different flavors on it.

CHILD: And sprinkles that pour off the top like rainbow rain!

Call it improv, family-style. When you adopt a 'yes, and' approach with your kids, you encourage their creativity and show them that you are present, listening and engaged. It's a tactic that can work wonders – even in those more serious exchanges where you are decidedly opposed to what your child is proposing.

The power lies with the *and*. It says, "I accept your idea, and I'm going to build on it." *And* allows you to expand on that 'yes' and shape the outcome of an exchange in a collaborative way.

There's a whole psychological theory that supports this "yes brain" philosophy. Simply put, when we hear "no," we tend to fall into a reactive state, often experiencing many of the same sensations we feel when threatened. In contrast, parenting with a "yes" approach results in more balanced, curious and receptive thinking on the part of the child – while still providing structure and discipline.

A yes-focused communication style encourages a child's ability to view the world as a place where they can thrive – relying on their own ability to be balanced, resilient, insightful and empathetic.

It's not about permissiveness. It's about creating optimism through the way we communicate. "Yes" keeps positivity alive.

## GIVE "NO" THE DAY OFF.

Let's imagine how "yes, and" might work in a non-goofing-around, typical mealtime encounter. First, the historic and popular "no" approach:

SCENE 2 (the kitchen):

> ARTICULATE CHILD: Hey Mom! Guess what? I really, really hate brussels sprouts. How about I just have a pile of Tootsie Rolls for dinner?

> OLD YOU: *Absolutely not!* Your teeth will rot right out of your head. Now eat up.

> ARTICULATE CHILD: I feel as if you are overreacting. In protest, I refuse to eat anything.

Versus taking the "yes, and" approach:

SCENE 2 REVISED (the kitchen):

ARTICULATE CHILD: Hey Mom! Guess what? I really, really hate brussels sprouts. How about I just have a pile of Tootsie Rolls for dinner?

NEW, EVOLVED YOU: Yes! In fact, I think we should make a Tootsie Roll casserole with whipped cream topping. Wouldn't that be amazing? But after that, we'll probably need to head straight to the dentist to have all your cavities filled. I'll drive and you pay.

ARTICULATE CHILD (shocked/confused and successfully distracted from the topic): Whaaaaa?

NEW EVOLVED YOU: (whispers to audience) *Psych!!*

See what new, evolved you did right there? You yes-anded your way out of a potential power struggle. You showed you were listening, acknowledged your child's creativity, added to it, and then directed the discussion – all while imparting a solid lesson on oral hygiene. Good going! Also, cue the Tony Awards, because wow on that performance!

## AMPLIFY YOUR EFFORTS.

☐ **Let your kids in on the "yes, and" secret.** Plan improv sessions where the whole family shares the fun – taking turns building stories with the goal of being as outrageous as possible.

☐ **Challenge yourself to substitute "no" with "yes, and" for one day and see what happens.** Embrace opportunities to think, "How can I make this work?" before nixing new ideas.

# RESOURCES:

Jain R: *Use the secret improv comedy in everyday parenting*, 2017. Available at: https://gozen.com/improv-comedy-and-parenting/

Siegel D: *The yes brain approach to parenting and life*, 2017. Available at: https://health.usnews.com/wellness/for-parents/articles/2017-11-29/the-yes-brain-approach-to-parenting-and-life.

Simons S: *How improv's golden rule can help you better connect with your kids*, 2017. Available at: www.fatherly.com/love-money/relationships/parenting-strategies-advice/improv-golden-rule-parents-greatest-asset/.

# NOTES:

# 9

# JUST *Breathe*

"When I was in third grade, my teacher invited the class to the carpet to lie on our backs. In a soothing voice, she encouraged us to close our eyes and place our hands on our bellies. 'Breathe in through your nose and notice how your hands rise and fall as your belly fills,' she said. I remember thinking this was the dumbest thing ever—until a few minutes later when I heard her softly calling my name. I had fallen asleep!"

This is how your day is unfolding: Your toddler refuses to nap. The phone is ringing, your toilet is clogged (coincidentally, the aforementioned toddler is missing a shoe) and you're late picking up your daughter from school. Suffice it to say somebody is about to have a meltdown, and this time that somebody is well over the age of 25. Even small annoyances like traffic or breaking a glass can add up to make a day especially difficult. The same thing happens to kids, too!

So, what can you – and your keyed-up child – do to calm down when things feel like they're spinning out of control? A simple, effective place to start is to *just breathe*. Yes, deep breathing can help both kids and parents to calm down.

But isn't breathing automatic, you ask? Well, yes—and no. When we're stressed or anxious, our breathing changes. Instead of inhaling and exhaling naturally, we take shorter, quicker

breaths—which may intensify panic and exacerbate whatever problem we're facing. That goes for both kids *and* adults.

Physiologically, deep breathing, as opposed to the shallower breaths we typically take, builds flexibility and resilience. As with any "exercise," the more you practice, the more your lung capacity increases—enabling even deeper breathing.

The science is certainly compelling. According to experts, calm breathing:

- Slows the heart rate and reduces anxiety
- Increases focus and attention
- Relieves pain
- Increases blood flow
- Improves posture
- Detoxifies the body
- Cultivates inner wisdom and strength
- Enhances creativity

Children who have been traumatized, have learning disabilities, get anxious easily, or suffer from other sensory issues are especially susceptible to stress reactions. Calm breathing activates a child's parasympathetic nervous system—minimizing defensiveness and helping them relax. Such mindful breathing integrates the body and mind—enabling humans to soothe, support or energize themselves.

Bottom line: Teaching kids to be aware of their breath and, by extension, their moods and feelings, can go a long way toward preventing disruptive behavior. And the other bottom line – modeling deep breathing can both help you and show your kids when, why and how deep breathing is a good idea.

## IN THROUGH THE NOSE, OUT THROUGH THE MOUTH.

It sounds silly to suggest "teaching" children what would seem the most natural of human functions. But *mindful* breathing takes practice. Introducing children to it at an early age is a wonderful gift we can bestow.

Calm, mindful breathing shifts a child's mind-body state—enabling them to become more aware, gain control, and manage their feelings. Not surprisingly, it has the same effect on adults. Bonus: when we're feeling calm, aware and in control, we also tend to be more thoughtful and kinder.

Try this:

☐ **With younger children, explain that calm, slow breathing can help them feel better when they are worried, anxious, or upset.** Teach them to breathe in slowly through their nose for about 4 seconds, then hold for 1-2 seconds. Next, exhale through their mouth for at least 4 seconds. Wait a few seconds before taking in the next deep breath.

☐ **For teens, wait 5-7 seconds between breaths.**

☐ **For all, repeat 5-10 times.**

## AMPLIFY YOUR EFFORTS.

☐ **Get your belly involved!** Have your child place one hand on their chest and the other on their abdomen, then breathe deeply, making sure the diaphragm – not the chest – expands. Think of the way newborns breathe. Try doing 6-10 per minute for 1-2 minutes a day. Try it together!

☐ **Blow some bubbles!** This well-loved pastime is an ideal way to have fun and teach little ones deep breathing skills. Encourage slow exhales that make for excellent bubble production. Then wait a beat before the next dip of the wand.

☐ **Yoga and meditation.** Check out the resources in your community – including your closest Parks and Recreation department – to see if they offer classes for kids or parent/child together. There are also yoga/meditation websites specifically designed for young children. Check out https://www.mindyeti.com for some great ones.

☐ **Practice.** Children who are anxious can learn to deep breathe before entering a potentially stressful situation or thinking about traumatic events. Practicing what to do can give your child a tool for managing their stress, no matter when or how it occurs.

Reinforce with children that calm breathing is something they can do anytime, anywhere. It can be their (and your) secret tool against all things scary, upsetting or overwhelming.

# RESOURCES:

American Academy of Pediatrics, Section on Integrative Medicine: *Just breathe: the importance of meditation breaks for kids, 2017.* Available at: www.healthychildren.org/English/healthy-living/ emotional-wellness/Pages/Just-Breathe-The-Importance-of-Meditation-Breaks-for-Kids.aspx.

Babies to Bookworms: *15 of the best yoga books for kids,* 2018. Available at: https://www.Babiestobookworms. com/2018/01/11/15-of-the-best-yoga-books-for-kids/

Integrated Learning Centers: *Breathing exercises for sensory defensive and anxious kids,* 2016. Available at: www.ilslearningcorner. com/2016-10-breathing-exercises-sensory-defensive-kids/.

Move With Me Administration: *4 breathing exercises for kids,* 2014. Available at: www.move-with-me.com/video/4-breathing-exercises-for-kids/. (video. Not hyperlinked).

Verissimo A. (2020). *Mindfulness for kids: 12 calming exercises to teach your child.* Available at: www.connecticutchildrens.org/ coronavirus/resilience-is-mindfulness-calming-exercises-for-kids/

# NOTES:

# 10
# *Watch* YOUR (BODY) LANGUAGE

"I didn't fully understand my 'laser eyes' super powers until my son hit his pre-teen years. I quickly realized I had to become more mindful of my approach, aware of not only what I was saying but how I was saying it, or I risked shutting down those really important conversations and questions. I practiced using my 'soft eyes,' relaxed body language, and a softer tone of voice, which encouraged him to relax and speak more freely about things. I found that completely eliminating eye contact was the best way for me to broach the most sensitive topics with him. Conversations were easier and flowed naturally in the car or on a walk. I'm happy to say, for the most part, I've finally learned to tame those laser eyes."

If tweens or teens live under your roof, you're probably on to many of the techniques they employ to communicate without actually speaking to you.

An abridged English translator:

- **The Dramatic Eye Roll: "This conversation is ridiculous and, also, my life is unfair."** *(According to the dictionary, eye rolling for English-speaking people can indicate disbelief, annoyance, exasperation, or disdain.)*

- **The Shoulder Shrug:** "It would be a challenge for me to care less about what you're saying right now. It really would." *(The shoulder shrug generally indicates aloofness, indifference, or uncertainty.)*

- **The Crossed Arms with a Side Order of Scowl:** "I'm still not interested in listening to you. And on top of that, I'm highly annoyed." *(Crossed arms are a defensive gesture. Defense against discomfort, shyness, insecurity, or feeling offended. If the fists are also clenched, then the crossed arms posture indicates hostility.)*

- **The Head Shake/Pffft Combo:** "How is it that I, a young person, know so much more about life than you, an old person?" *(The transverse head shake indicates disagreement in many cultures, while "Pfft" is used to show a lack of interest in another or looking down on another person.)*

As adults, we recognize the meaning of these gestures because, let's be real, we pulled them on *our* parents. We may use them still, and as our parenting evolves, we tend to add new ones, like the finger wag or those dreaded 'laser eyes.' And, of course, body language and gestures may have different meanings across cultures.

Research shows that up to 55 percent of what we absorb from or communicate to others is achieved through body language, 38 percent through tone of voice, and just seven percent from actual words. Body language is powerful stuff, so it's important that we harness gestures and body postures to help communicate the important messages we really want our kids to hear. Keep in mind, too, that the same body language signs can have different meanings in different cultures.

## START WITH SOFT EYES.

You read that right. "Soft eyes" are a real thing – and a helpful tool for communicating more openly with anyone. The term refers to relaxing your gaze – and your mind along with it – to allow yourself to become open and take in a larger picture (as opposed to the 'hard' gaze you might need to, say, thread a needle). When talking with children, looking at them with soft, loving eyes shows kindness. It expresses less judgement, helps alleviate tension and promotes a feeling of calm – all great things for getting a message across the right way.

Other positive body language tips for communicating with kids:

- [ ] **Talk to them on their level**. Literally. Crouch, squat, or sit down at kid-height. This takes away the intimidation factor of towering over your child.

- [ ] **Watch your face**. Be aware of your expression and adjust accordingly. Smiles communicate encouragement, but that may not *always* be your goal – for instance, with the toddler who just loaded your dishwasher with pretzels. Sure, it's funny, but you don't want it happening again, so strive to keep your expression neutral when in discipline mode.

- [ ] **Uncross your arms**. You'll appear far less "judgy" and far more accepting.

- [ ] **Look them in the eyes**. And sometimes don't. You make the call: a direct-in-the-eyes gaze (even a soft one!) can help impart an urgent message, while avoiding eye contact and casually talking can sometimes help get your child (especially a teen) to open up.

- [ ] **Give plenty of high-fives, fist bumps, and thumbs ups**. They're encouraging, supportive and celebratory, *so don't hold back!*

## AMPLIFY YOUR EFFORTS.

The ability to pick up on what others are telling us through non-verbal cues is pivotal to developing good social skills and gaining acceptance from others. We've got to be able to recognize the difference between boring somebody to tears and genuinely captivating them!

One way to help kids develop their ability to read body language is by sharing pictures of people demonstrating a variety of facial expressions and asking your child to identify the possible emotions.

Got a group of kids? Try modifying a game like Telephone: instead of passing along a word or phrase, have the kids choose an emotion/expression that gets passed down the line and see how accurate they are when it gets to the last kid.

# RESOURCES:

Gamzo M: *10 Essential verbal communication skills that will make you a better parent*, 2015. Available at: https://afineparent.com/b-positive/non-verbal-communication-skills.html

Natural Parent Magazine: *7 Body language tips to communicate better with your child*. N. D. Available at: www.thenaturalparentmagazine.com/7-body-language-tips-communicate-better-child/.

Parvez H: *Body language: Crossing the arms meaning*. 2021. Available at: www.psychomechanics.com/body-language-crossing-arms/

Purvis A: *Starting small: eye contact*. Karen Purvis Institute for Child Development, 2019. Available at: www.child.tcu.edu/eye-contact/#sthash. fKsqd2kCdpbs.

Raising Children. Net: *Nonverbal communication: body language and tone of voice*. Available at: https://www.raisingchildren.net.au/toddlers/connecting-communicating/ nonverbal-communication

# NOTES:

# 11

## CULTIVATE *Wonder*

> "I will never forget taking my daughter camping for the first time. Everything from setting up the tent to fishing in the lake and splashing in the mud was a brand-new experience for her. The glee she felt was contagious!"

We throw the words "awesome" and "amazing" around an awful lot in our little corner of the world, but how often do we really, truly mean them? It seems the older we get, the more our sense of wonder dampens – as if we've seen it all before and none of it is really a big deal. Blazing pink and orange sunsets? Pretty, but…. Mozart's Piano Concerto #21? Meh. Giant redwood trees? Aren't there, like, three trillion trees in the world?

Small children, on the other hand, seem to approach the world with less of a stifled yawn and more of a the-hills-are-alive-with-the-sound-of-music-full-twirl-in-an-alpine-meadow sort of enthusiasm. For them, everything is new, and here's something cool: One of the most amazing parts of spending time with a child is the opportunity to experience our everyday activities from a brand-new perspective – theirs. Imagine feeling the grass between your toes, grabbing a fistful of puppy fur or tasting ice cream for the very first time. It all falls squarely into the "wow!" category.

As kids grow, that phase of innocent discovery often dims into an "I'm bored" appearance. Let's work toward cultivating and keeping a sense of wonder alive – for our kids and ourselves. Why? Because viewing the world in this way:

- Broadens social connections
- Stimulates curiosity and expands creativity
- Leads to kindness and generosity
- Makes us more grateful
- Improves the immune system
- Reduces anxiety and depression

Living with a sense of wonder just plain makes life more enjoyable, and if we can slow down and relish in these moments with kids, the experience is that much more wonderful.

## SCHEDULE SOME AWESOME.

Tapping into wonder doesn't require a monumental effort, nor do we need to go very far to find it.

☐ **Take an awe walk.** Yep, it's a real thing. Turn off your cell phone and step outside. Even a stroll in your neighborhood or an outside area offers endless opportunities to cultivate wonder. Examine the sky and the clouds. Collect leaves, rocks or sticks and take some time to inspect them. Talk about how bugs and animals might use these items.

☐ **If you can, travel.** You don't necessarily have to go far. Search for wide open spaces, tall trees, soaring mountain peaks. Skyscrapers, cavernous stadiums, the glowing harvest moon – what's not to drop your jaw at?

☐ **Embrace music and art.** The sights. The sounds. The bottomless well of human talent that surrounds us. Explore listening to new styles of music or take a trip to an art museum and feast your eyes. Appreciate and discuss the effort behind the work even when it's not your favorite.

☐ **Focus on the microscopic.** Examining flowers and the tiny insects that gather on them is a fun way to talk about colors, shapes, sounds and textures.

☐ **Play with science.** Grab a book on science experiments from the children's section of the library and spend an afternoon blowing your mind.

☐ **Read inspiring books and explore websites** – about larger-than-life people, adventures or events.

☐ **"Wonder" the aisles at the grocery store.** Look for interesting produce you've never seen before. Smell it, touch it, name the colors. Make up new names for what you find!

Cultivating wonder creates opportunities for connection with the children in our lives while making everyday life more interesting. If *you* take the time to relish the moment, you'll likely notice your kids do, too.

## AMPLIFY YOUR EFFORTS.

For teens, photographing nature or drawing can be wonderful gateways to appreciating the world around them. For the more scientific types, explore the possibility of joining a science club or robotics group. Figuring out how things work is part of wonder too.

For parents, try to focus less on rushing around with your head down and more on paying attention and being in the moment. SEE what's around you. Engage all your senses and share that with a child. The world – and the future – needs their sense of wonder.

---

## RESOURCES:

Greater Good in Action: *Awe Walk*. Available at: https://ggia.berkeley.edu/practice/awe_walk

Parent.co: *How awe transforms us and how to create more of it for your kids*, 2017. Available at: https://www.parent.com/blogs/conversations/the-power-of-awe-why-our-children-need-more-and-how-to-ensure-they-get-it.

Smith J: *The benefits of feeling awe.* Greater Good Magazine, 2016. Available at: www.ggia.berkeley.edu/article/item/the_benefits_of_feeling_awe.

Tix A: Nurturing Awe in Kids. *Psychology Today.* 2015. Available at: www.psychologytoday.com/us/blog/the-pursuit-peace/201509/nurturing-awe-in-kids.

_____

# NOTES:

# 12

# WAKE UP THEIR *Inner Artist*

"Stories, poems and music were instilled in me from the get-go: by my piano-playing Pops who would alter lyrics of favorite songs to see if I was paying attention, by my sister who would pause before turning the page to ask, 'what do you think will happen next?' (and actually listen to my answer), and by my brother who drew self-portraits with sidewalk chalk and asked for my artistic observations. It's how I learned to connect, understand, and appreciate – myself, the people I knew, and everything else. None of my family used the arts to make a living, but when one or more of us were doing something related to the arts, we were at our best. Most open. Most generous. Most playful. Most human."

You've got the parenting basics covered. When your kids are hungry, you feed them. When they cry, you comfort them. You put shoes on their little feet and hats on their fuzzy heads, and make sure they're tucked into bed before 8 p.m. It's all important stuff.

Parenting is in the details, details, details. But once kids' basic needs are met, what's next? Plenty, of course. But how about this: What feeds their creativity? What fuels their spirit? And, why does it matter?

Philip Pullman, an award-winning author of children's books – and apparently a reflective type – has observed that "Children need art and stories and poems and music as much as they need love and food and fresh air and play."

The arts ground and connect us in unique and wonderful ways, providing opportunities to observe the world – and life – through another person's eyes. And art is right there in both the planned and unexpected details: A song that's like an instant time machine back to middle school. The Michelangelo masterpiece that simultaneously makes your jaw drop and your arm hairs stand up. (He painted *that*? On the *ceiling*?) Chalk-drawn street art, an expertly crafted sandcastle, a poem or book that somehow feels laser-focused right at YOU. Art is endlessly inserting itself in our lives. As a parent, why not reach out, grab those opportunities and share the magic with your kids?

If science and math are more your priority, know this: there's measurable value behind all this art talk. Arts education – and involvement in the arts – actually helps kids learn and perform better in every discipline and deliver higher scores in math, reading, cognitive ability, critical thinking and verbal skills. They also play a key role in the development of motor skills, language, decision making, and visual learning.

Plus – get this – making art (and that can be in a variety of forms – including music and dance) helps kids process trauma and build emotional resilience.

Best of all, the chance to create, learn about, and appreciate art makes for some well-rounded kids—and our world can sure use that!

## SCULPT A PLAN.

Art is free. Although many people may think learning or engaging in the arts requires money, that is not necessarily true. Art and creativity are everywhere, and in countless forms, so don't let your wallet hold you back. We're talking symphonies and bucket drummers, fine art and street art, film, theater and improv, woodworking and paper crafts, photography in museums and photo projects on Instagram, long novels and short stories. Just pick something and dive in.

Need some more inspiration?

☐ **Start a craft closet** (or drawer, or even an over-sized plastic bin). Stock it with empty paper towel rolls and construction paper, scrap paper and old magazines, ribbons and buttons, glitter and beads – essentially anything that stands half a chance of being glued to something else. Add markers, crayons, glue sticks and safety scissors and declare your "creation station" open for business. Frame and display some of your kids' favorite creations.

☐ **Fill another bin with an assortment of dress-up options**: capes, fairy wings, old Halloween costumes, hats and shoes, jewelry. Let the creative play commence.

☐ **Take field trips.** Head out to a local art museum and spark discussion about the pieces you encounter. Ask your kids questions: "What do you think the artist was feeling when they created it – and how does it make you feel?" "What are the materials and colors used – and why do you think the artist chose them?"

☐ **Let teens, and even younger kids, call most of the shots on decorating their rooms.** Maybe a chalkboard wall or funky new paint color can be a backdrop for them to display their talents and creative ideas. On a smaller scale, making memory books of their activities, tie-dyeing tee shirts or displaying their collections can be fun. It also shows that you value their efforts.

☐ **Look for free (or cheap) concerts and musical performances** in your community. Check out theater offerings at the local high school and encourage kids who are old enough to get involved. And take full advantage of your local library: story time, events, art displays and – oh yes – books!

☐ **Plan a family photography show.** Select a theme (nature, animals, or architecture for instance), then print and frame some of your favorites. Frames are cheap at garage sales or thrift stores.

## AMPLIFY YOUR EFFORTS.

Many schools are under-funded or have been forced to eliminate or scale back arts and music programs. Put the power of volunteerism to work and start an art or music education program at your child's school. This can be in addition to existing art and music classes, offering expanded learning with hands-on application. (Check out programs like this for inspiration: www.musicworkshopedu.org.)

And remember this: Not every kid will be lit up by the arts, but every kid deserves a chance to discover what lights their inner fire. Let's give them all the opportunity to flip that switch.

## RESOURCES:

Artword Archive: *How to get your kids interested in art*, 2019. Available at: https://www.artworkarchive.com/blog/how-to-get-your-kids-interested-in-art

Flowers J: *Art heals! How the arts build resilient brains and bodies*, 2017. www.acesconnection.com/blog/art-heals-how-the-arts-build-resilient-brains-and-bodies?reply=470108789082755268.

Frey S: *Art appreciation helps young children learn to think and express ideas*, 2015. Available at: www.edsource.org/2015/art-appreciation-helps-young-children-learn-to-think-and-express-ideas/77734.

Pullman P: *Children need art and stories and poems and music as much as they need love and food and fresh air and play*, 2012. Available at: www.astridlindgrenmemorialaward.wordpress.com/2015/12/17/children-need-art-and-stories-and-poems-and-music-as-much-as-they-need-love-and-food-and-fresh-air-and-play/.

Robinson K Sir, Aronica L: *What happens to student behavior when schools prioritize art*, 2018. Available at: www.kqed.org/mindshift/50874/what-happens-to-student-behavior-when-schools-prioritize-art.

---

# NOTES:

# 13

# *Get* COMFORTABLE BEING UNCOMFORTABLE

"I remember how hard it was for me to talk about the onset of puberty with my oldest daughter. She needed information but froze up and yelled "Mommm! Stop!" whenever I tried to talk about it with her. Something I finally learned in raising three kids is that the less of a big deal I make about awkward subjects, the less of a big deal it will be for them. By taking this approach, I've been able to develop relationships with my kids where they come to me about things I wouldn't have dreamed of talking about with my own parents."

Puberty. Relationships. Sex. Drugs. Violence. Death. Sexually transmitted infections.

Does anybody actually *look forward* to discussing these sorts of topics with their children? If you answer "yes", please consider hosting a seminar for the rest of us. For any number of reasons, broaching these and other uncomfortable issues can land well outside the comfort zone of most parents.

But we need to talk about them. As parents, sharing insights on hard-hitting topics is an opportunity to express our values and appropriate personal experiences as well as ensure that kids hear facts, not rumors. Open communication begins with you.

Studies show that teens who feel connected to their parents report less cannabis use and may delay sexual activity until they

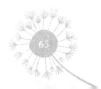

are older. One key to building that connection is a comfort level in discussing difficult topics without fear of rejection or a parental freak out. Granted, getting some kids to share their deepest thoughts and concerns – or even just getting them to tell you about their day – can be difficult. On the flip side, others share so much you may sometimes want to tune out because of your own discomfort. Parents of these kids: consider yourself lucky.

The moral of all this? Your willingness to start a discussion – and keep the doors open – on any subject is key to building trust and a strong family dynamic, where your children will feel comfortable coming to *you* with problems.

## BUCKLE UP AND JUMP IN.

☐ **First, check your facts.** If you aren't fully educated about the information you plan to share, start with some research. Real-life case in point: a well-meaning grandmother who, in explaining the evils of drug use to a pre-teen, mixed up the side of effects of LSD and cannabis. Her intentions were good, but her credibility was zero.

☐ **Plan the when and where.** Timing is everything. If there's something you know you want to discuss with your child, you can increase your comfort level and chance for success by getting the setting right. Some popular places for encouraging information sharing include the car (you're stuck together anyway and eye contact is optional, so you may make some real headway), a hike or neighborhood walk, around the dinner table or at a family meeting. Beware, though, that choosing the car may make some kids feel trapped, especially if that is the place you always choose for hard conversations.

☐ **Take cues from a TV show or movie.** If you're watching together as a family, the subject matter may provide the perfect opportunity to bring up a topic in a natural way.

☐ **Use books.** There are many resources for introducing children to difficult subjects through narrative stories. Fair warning though: you can't expect to adequately address puberty by throwing "What's Going on Down There?" at your middle-schooler and then exiting the room. Some topics call for face-to-face Q and A.

☐ **Don't lecture.** Instead, communicate. Aim for a healthy discussion that allows for thoughtful questions and answers on both sides.

☐ **Be a good listener.** Listen with the goal of guiding – not controlling – your kids. Hear them out and ask questions that lead you to a better understanding of what they are trying to tell – or ask – you.

## AMPLIFY YOUR EFFORTS.

Still struggling with getting a discussion rolling? Try printing out some questions or topics you can pull out of a paper bag and discuss. Better yet, try and get your kids to write their own questions. They may find that approach easier than having to speak the words out loud.

## RESOURCES:

Family First, LLC: *Hard topics to talk about for kids*, 2019. Available at: www.imom.com/5-hard-topics-to-talk-about-for-kids/#. W1t38tJKg2w.

GracieX: *How I raised teenagers who tell me everything---even when it's hard*, 2019. Available at: www.mindbodygreen.com/0-22738/how-i-raised-teenagers-who-tell-me-everything-even-when-its-hard. html.

National Society for the Prevention of Cruelty to Children (NSPCC): *Talking about difficult topics*, 2019. Available at: www.nspcc.org.uk/preventing-abuse/keeping-children-safe/ talking-about-difficult-topics/.

## NOTES:

# 14

# *Connect* WITH YOUR TERRIFIC TEEN

"Watching our teens graduate from high school brought me to tears. I was thinking 'how did we get here when they were so little just a short time ago?' We had so many things to teach them and protect them from and now they are about to go out on their own."

The years from 12 to 21 are marvelous to behold. Not only are there the changes in body shape, size, and function, but also changes in thinking, acting, and relating to other people. There will be days when you will marvel at the poised, intelligent and articulate 16-year-old who just yesterday was afraid go to intermediate school. There will be moments when you will wonder when your six-foot young man body-snatched the adorable kid who used to live in the room at the end of the hall.

There will most definitely be times when you will search for the strength to graciously navigate the miraculous but not-for-the-faint-of-heart journey from your kids' childhood to young adulthood. No question about it: getting through the teenage years will earn you the right to wear the (slightly askew) crown of parenthood.

So what, exactly, is the deal with teenagers? As in: what is actually going on in their heads? Turns out, a lot. The brain's prefrontal cortex, which drives logical thinking – and that famous "executive functioning" we hear a lot about – doesn't fully develop until about age 25. That leaves the amygdala – part of the brain in charge of processing emotions – to do some heavy lifting. As a result, teenagers don't always *think* so much as they *feel* and *act*. They can be complex, transparent, naïve, moody, kind, mature or painfully immature, impulsive, thoughtful, transparent, compassionate, mind-bogglingly self-centered, industrious, lazy...the list goes on. And some days, you'll get to witness all the above before they even take off for school in the morning.

What we consider the "teen" development phase encompasses more or less nine years – from about 12 to 21 years of age. Developmental psychologists divide the time into early, middle, and late phases. The early teen focusing on the physical changes is much different from the middle teen working on establishing a self and making independent decisions. The late teen typically is thinking about jobs, more permanent relationships, advanced education, and living away from home.

It all adds up to what can be a whole lot of emotional ups and downs for everyone. The issues often revolve around letting them make decisions and take risks but stay safe at the same time. There's a good chance you'll spend more time worrying about your kids now than you ever have as they push forward toward adulthood. Prepare to be firm but flexible as you all navigate this inevitable stage. Just as with younger kids, your approaches at each level will need to change.

## EARN YOUR PARENTING CROWN.

The bond you have built with your kid over the years will be your best tool in keeping your relationship afloat during the teenage years. As their needs change, you'll need to gear up to adapt right along with them.

10 Do's and a Don't for setting a positive vibe for the teen years:

☐ **DO set clear expectations. This should be a continuation from early childhood. Consequences should be clear. For example, if your child wants permission to go out with** friends, you can reasonably ask them to give you three pieces of information: 1) Where are you going? 2) Who are you going with? 3) What time will you be home?

☐ **DO follow through consistently** when a rule – such as a curfew violation – is broken.

☐ **DO carve out time together.** Even a few minutes in the morning or at the end of the day goes a long way toward keeping a pulse on what's happening in your kid's life. Continue eating meals together when you can and strive for one or two outings together a week – even short ones.

☐ **DO show flexibility in negotiating non-safety related rules.** This might include how they choose to wear their hair, what music they listen to or anything that that does not pose a legitimate threat to their physical or emotional safety. This helps kids build solid decision-making skills.

☐ **DON'T take everything personally.** Fighting and arguing are common as teens practice their reasoning skills and push for independence. This probably isn't about you.

☐ **DO stay involved in their lives.** Make it a point to know their friends and communicate with their friends' parents, show up for their activities, support their interests and communicate with their teachers.

☐ **DO encourage healthy behaviors.** Eating well, getting exercise, staying away from alcohol and drugs are all good choices. Talk with your kids about why these things matter.

☐ **DO continue to involve teens in family activities.** Allowing them to bring a friend along helps!

☐ **DO keep your promises,** model good behavior and always keep communication lines open.

☐ **DO tell them you love them** – and demonstrate it – every single day.

## AMPLIFY YOUR EFFORTS.

It is the hard truth that many kids will give their parents genuine reason for concern. If you've ever reflected on your own teenage years and admitted "I was awful. What in the world was I thinking?" you may have been one of them.

Your teenager may be moody but shouldn't live in their room 23 hours of the day. Teen behaviors that may fall outside the realm of "normal" and inching into dangerous territory include: repeated drinking or drug use, sexual activity (dependent on age and situation), getting into fights, criminal acts, skipping school or self-harming. Likewise, signs of eating disorders, depression or anxiety call for action. Do not wait to call for help on such issues. School counselors, your primary care provider, or a help line can be ready resources for you.

You should expect arguing, but not violent aggression or constant conflict. You can anticipate most teens will try alcohol or smoking at some point, but regular drinking and drug use are unhealthy behaviors regardless of age. It can be tough to define the line between what is and is not of concern when it comes to this developmental stage.

If you are a single parent, this is a time to try to collaborate with the teen's other parent or people whom you trust and rely upon. Consistency regarding expectations is important and sharing observations may be essential.

Be diligent, but don't hesitate to call in the experts – a doctor, therapist or counselor – when you feel out of your league.

# RESOURCES:

Davis JL: *10 Parenting tips for raising teenagers.*
Available at: www.webmd.com/parenting/
features/10-parenting-tips-for-raising-teenagers#1

Davis JL: Teenagers: Why do they rebel? WebMD Archives.
Available at: https://www.webmd.com/parenting/features/
teenagers-why-do-they-rebel#1

Garey J: *10 Tips for parenting your pre-teen*, n.d. WebMD
Archives. Available at: https://www.webmd.com/parenting/
features/10-tips-parenting-your-preteen#1

Markham L: *Gameplan for positive parenting your teen.* Available at:
www.ahaparenting.com/ages-stages/teenagers/parenting-teens

# NOTES:

# 15
## GIVE YOURSELF A *Break*

"Parenting is rewarding, but it definitely comes with struggles. Despite our best intentions, we make mistakes. A phrase I used with my toddler on especially difficult or emotional days – when voices were raised or snippy answers given – was 'Although we get frustrated with each other, we still love each other.' Naming the emotion and refocusing on love helped both of us. My son would usually give me a big smile when he heard this and I would feel as if I had regained some control. It's normal to struggle, but I learned to be patient with myself and let some things go. As a parent, it's important to literally give yourself a break so you can focus on being you."

No parent is perfect. If any life experience is designed to make us question our competency on a daily basis, it's parenthood. You can read all the books and take all the classes and feed your kids healthy snacks. Still, you can be emotionally wrestled to the ground by a sassy six-year-old. How is that even possible?

The simple answer is: you're human. While the parenting journey can be oh-so-rewarding, it is also *long* and roller-coasterish. We yell, we say things we know we shouldn't or overreact to a situation. As long as you aren't causing actual physical or psychological harm to your children, it's the way you move forward *after* those moments of frustration that matter most.

On those occasions when you feel frustrated or overwhelmed, give yourself a moment to calm down. Take a deep breath and then, if the situation warrants it, apologize. It can be as simple as "I'm very sorry I spoke to you that way. I wish I had said _____. Let's start over."

Don't continue to make a big deal out of what you said or did, and don't be too hard on yourself over it. Simply own your actions, apologize and move on. In the process, you'll be teaching your kids healthy coping mechanisms that leave no room for negative self-talk for when they make their own mistakes.

## RECHARGE YOUR BATTERIES.

The emotional drain is real, as every parent knows. Being your best self requires regular time outs – the kind where caregivers get a chance to walk away from parenting duties, even if only for a few minutes or hours.

Some quick attitude pick-me-ups:

- [ ] **Meditate** to decrease stress and let go of distractions. This can be as basic as sitting in a quiet place, closing your eyes and focusing on breathing for several minutes. You can even try to take some deep breaths while waiting at a stoplight!

- [ ] **Take a walk around the block.** Or run. Fresh air and exercise are fantastic mind declutterers.

- [ ] **Sit in the sun.**

- [ ] **Call a friend.**

- [ ] **Write in a journal.** Or read a book.

- [ ] **Plan a vacation.** Positive anticipation of something great can breathe new life into your days.

- [ ] **Listen to music you love.**

- [ ] **Do something artsy-craftsy.** Concentrating on making something – with no pressure attached – is therapeutic.

- [ ] **Daydream.** About your future, your goals, or whatever relaxes you.

- [ ] **Hire a babysitter or plan to swap childcare time with a friend or relative** and take some time to do whatever you want to do!

## AMPLIFY YOUR EFFORTS.

First, know this: kids don't need "perfect" parents in order to grow up into super cool, happy, and thriving world citizens. And we certainly shouldn't expect perfection from our children, either. You just need to be *good enough*. And good enough parents still make mistakes.

That said, nobody wants to lose their temper with their children on a frequent basis. So, work to build awareness of the types of situations that cause you to become upset. Know what causes you stress, anticipate what might set you off, then make a concerted effort to prepare for – and be better in – those moments.

If you can't seem to find a way to calm yourself with regular breaks, ask for help from a mental health professional. You can't be the best for your children if you are not at your best for yourself.

---

# RESOURCES:

Bergen County Grief Counseling: *Self-care is important for parents,* 9/2019. Available at: http://www.bergencountygriefcounseling. com/index.php/blog/195-self-care-parents

Coyne M: *Why parental self-care is essential for children's emotional wellbeing.* Available at: https://www.alustforlife.com/mental-health/ children-and-adolescents/why-parental-self-care-is-essential-for-childrens-emotional-wellbeing

Gray P: *The good-enough parent is the best parent*, Dec. 22, 2015. Available at: www.psychologytoday.com/us/blog/freedom-learn/201512/the-good-enough-parent-is-the-best-parent.

Hilkey C: *Parents make mistakes too – how to apologize.* Available at: www.happilyfamily.com/parents-make-mistakes-how-to-apologize/.

Tyler T: *Packing our emotional first aid kit*, May, 2021. Girls Leadership. Available at: http://www.girlsleadership.org/author/takai-tyler

---

# NOTES:

# 16
## *Believe* IN THEM

"My son loves school and is a strong student, yet he always resists taking on challenging math and reading classes. We end up having lengthy discussions before he'll agree to try any new class situation. What I hear from him is: 'I might not be good enough.' 'Are any of my friends going to be there?' 'Can I be reassigned to a different level if I can't do it?' 'Is the teacher nice?' He always needs that vote of confidence before he makes a decision, so I work really hard to make sure he knows that I believe in his abilities and that if he doesn't try, he'll never learn what he's truly capable of."

*ehind every child who believes in themself is a parent who believed in them first.* We would have come up with that line ourselves if somebody hadn't beaten us to it. Here's why: Every kid needs at least one cheerleader and from day one, parents, that cheerleader should be you.

A key ingredient in raising kids with strong self-esteem is making sure they know how much we believe in them. Confidence helps form a foundation for healthy relationships throughout life and equips children (and adults) to overcome setbacks, giving them the perspective to accept disappointments as both a source of insight and a normal part of life.

Kids – especially young ones – take their cues from their parents.

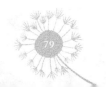

You're like a mirror; their sense of identity is largely a reflection of how *you* look at them. You are uniquely positioned to instill the powerful sense of belonging and safety kids need to truly be themselves – free to discover their own special qualities and skills. By the way, you're also the number one candidate to teach your kids how to "look on the bright side" or "turn lemons into lemonade" – a mindset that is consistent with hope, possibility, and confidence.

The pride you express in your kids – both directly to them and to others (make sure they eavesdrop on some controlled bragging from time-to-time) – helps develop passion and enthusiasm for what they enjoy and excel at. Most of us have figured out by now that giving every kid a trophy for just showing up somewhere doesn't build them into better people. But encouragement, support, reassurance, and praise for hard work does. So, encourage them to try new things. Encourage them to challenge themselves. Encourage them to dream – and follow those dreams.

As the saying goes, it's not about winning or losing – but how we play the game. Parenting – and life – are much more enjoyable when we celebrate effort instead of outcomes.

## YOU CAN DO IT!

The work of helping kids build self-esteem can be one of most satisfying responsibilities of parenthood.

Some ways to start:

- [ ] **Be generous with praise and sparse with criticism.** Strive for a ratio of 10 positives to every negative.

- [ ] **Speak politely to them – and others.**

- [ ] **Always keep the lines of communication open.**

- [ ] **Tell them that you believe in them. Then show them.**

- [ ] **Guide them in turning frustrations into learning opportunities (that's the lemons into lemonade bit referenced earlier).**

☐ **Let them know that they're valued.**

☐ **Help them set attainable goals.** And help them find a coach, tutor, or mentor in the community if that goal is a bit of a stretch.

☐ **Use visualization exercises to help them "see" themselves as successful.**

☐ **Listen to them!**

## AMPLIFY YOUR EFFORTS.

Inspiration is everywhere! Reading stories about people who have overcome challenges and doubts can help build the knowledge that success is waiting for those who believe in themselves and are ready to put the work in. So, head to the library to look for biographies of famous or successful people—especially those who have overcome long odds. Read and discuss those journeys with your kids. Then help them define "success" in their own terms—and set goals to achieve it in pursuits big and small.

As teens approach high school graduation, they'll need your support as much as ever. Big decisions – about college, career options, and learning how to function fully as an adult – are just around the corner. There's no one-size-fits-all approach to growing up and establishing autonomy. Be sure they know you're behind them and that the doors are open for them to change course or explore new opportunities.

---

# RESOURCES:

Foster BJ: *Jim Valvano and the power of believing in your kids*, 2018. Available at: http://www.allprodad.com/jim-valvano-and-the-power-of-believing-in-your-kids/.

Inspired by family: The power of believing in your kids, 2018. Available at: https://www.inspiredbyfamilymag.com/2018/08/08/believing-in-your-kids/

Myers RC: 11 Tips on building self-esteem in children. 2020. Available at: https://www.todaysparent.com/family/parenting/how-to-build-your-childs-self-esteem

Newman S: *How allowing your children to fail helps them succeed*, 2015. Psychology Today. Available at: www.psychologytoday.com/us/blog/singletons/201508/how-allowing-children-fail-helps-them-succeed

---

# NOTES:

# PART TWO

## CREATING STABILITY FOR THE FAMILY

Stability: The degree of predictability
and consistency in a child's social,
emotional and physical environment.[*]

A family is like a mobile – bending and gently twirling in the breeze, all the parts working together. Much like a mobile, maintaining a stable family environment requires the members to work together. Remove one part or add too much weight, and the whole structure loses its balance. In this section, we offer tips to help keep your family in balance – creating an environment where every member knows what to expect and can find satisfaction and comfort in that understanding.

Creating stability in a family means kids can expect social, emotional, and physical consistency from the adults they count on. That includes being

---

* Centers for Disease Control, National Center for Injury Prevention and Control, Division of Violence Prevention: Essentials for Childhood: Creating Safe, Nurturing Relationships and Environments for All Children, 2019

there – to tuck them in, cheer for them at soccer, help with home-work or walk them home from school. It also means creating routines for things like meals, sleep, and play. It's not always easy to pull off, but when all goes smoothly, it's a fantastic achievement. This section focuses on organizing the family for fun and stability.

# 17

# EAT DINNER *Together*

"I visit my niece every Tuesday evening to play, eat and read. It's my favorite night of the week! Spending this time together has really strengthened our relationship—and it's a lot of fun! Eating together as a family builds a sense of community and love."

Mealtime. It rolls around three times a day. It doesn't have to be fancy, beautiful, or even over-the-top delicious, but we've all got to eat. And, according to experts, the very best family meals are served up *together*.

Shared family meals have positive effects on the "spirit, brain and health of all family members," say the folks at *The Family Dinner Project*, a Harvard University-based nonprofit. Regular family meals (no matter what time of day), these experts have found, can lead to all sorts of bonuses for kids: higher grade-point averages, stronger self-esteem, and lower rates of substance abuse, teen pregnancy, eating disorders and depression.

More to the point, says Anne Fishel, co-founder of *The Family Dinner Project*, the "daily mealtime connection is like a seatbelt for traveling the potholed road of childhood and adolescence and all its possible risk behaviors." Now that's some good stuff!

A few other compelling reasons to make mealtime a family affair:

- Kids who share four or more weekly meals with their family do better on achievement tests than those who eat fewer meals together.

- Teens are more likely to talk to their parents during dinner than at any other time.
- Kids' thinking and linguistic development improve.
- Family meals contribute to healthy development even more than playtime or story time.
- Children who regularly eat with their family eat more vegetables and drink less soda.

Healthier nutrition. Healthier conversation. Healthier living and learning habits. They're all outcomes of regular family meals. If you're not currently eating together as a family, why not give it a try?

## DISH IT UP.

Family schedules are tricky to navigate (work, school, basketball, homework, music lessons, play practice, part-time jobs...we get it). Plan to stay flexible but firm in your commitment to make family dinner a priority. More meals together = more opportunities to turn down the volume on the rest of the day and focus on building a strong tradition every family member can look forward to, and kids can count on.

☐ **Set aside a few minutes on the weekend to plan meals for the upcoming week.**

☐ **Divvy up meal prep and clean-up responsibilities with designated assignments such as setting or clearing the table, assembling the salad, and loading the dishwasher.**

☐ **Turn off the TV and establish a no cell phone zone.**

☐ **Above all, mealtime should be a positive experience—so check disagreements and negativity at the door.**

## AMPLIFY YOUR EFFORTS.

☐ **Spice things up with a conversation starter.** Food for thought: If you could do anything you wanted all day, what would it be? Who was/is your favorite teacher, and why? What is something you're looking forward to right now? For more inspiration, head on over to *The Family Dinner Project*.

☐ **Pack up a picnic and relocate dinner to the backyard or park.**

☐ **Launch a new tradition (and make planning *way* easier) with a regular Tuesday Taco or Friday Pizza night.**

☐ **Assign each family member a night to plan and prepare a meal.**

☐ **Cook a meal together and then deliver or share it with a family which could use a hand.**

---

## RESOURCES:

Fishel AK: *The most important thing you can do with your kids? Eat dinner with them.* Available at: https://www.washingtonpost.com/posteverything/wp/2015/01/12/the-most-important-thing-you-can-do-with-your-kids-eat-dinner-with-them/

Jackson J & L: *Struggling at the family dinner table? How to come together and enjoy.* Connected Families. Available at: www.Connectedfamilies.org/family-mealtime/

McEntire T: *Why families should eat dinner together.* 2021. Available at: https://www.families.com/why-families-should-eat-dinner-together

Veling J: *Why families should eat dinner together* Active Kids Available at: https://www.activekids.com/parenting-and-family/articles/why-families-should-eat-dinner-together.

# NOTES:

# 18

## ROLL THE DICE FOR FAMILY
# Game Night

> "When I was growing up, my family engaged in regular game nights whenever we could. They were our best times together! We stopped being 'parents' and 'children' and we all became 'people' and relaxed. It was a great way to get to know my parents as people...and then beat them at cards without consequences!"

You've probably heard it many times before, but this bears repeating: *families who play together stay together*. Maybe that's an oversimplification. But it's a fact that time spent together – having *actual* fun – builds important family bonds.

Strong families are healthy families, where both kids and parents thrive. Carving out time to engage in positive activities together – such as a regular family game night – can be a giant step on the path to building a rock-solid family dynamic.

The lasting impact of healthy family activities on a child's development is overwhelming. Research shows that children whose families encourage open lines of communication and opportunities for interactive play reap life-changing benefits. Among them:

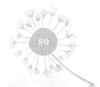

- Larger vocabularies
- Better motor skills
- Better school performance
- Improved reading scores
- Motivation to learn
- Stronger relationships with peers
- Enhanced problem-solving ability
- Learning to follow rules
- A healthier sense of well-being...and much more

For parents, game night presents an opportunity to launch a family tradition, create memories and practice positive role modeling skills. It is also a great time to begin teaching about following rules – for the game, for personal boundaries, and for the laws of society. Plus, you'll emerge as the Fun Captain of the family. Prepare for uplifted moods and lasting smiles all around.

## GET THE BALL (OR DICE) ROLLING.

☐ **Mark an "X" on your calendar,** let the kids know what's up and recruit them to help plan! Compile a list of potential games.

☐ **Plan to pair smaller children with older siblings or an adult to encourage teamwork** and even the playing field.

☐ **Make sure everyone understands that healthy competition is great, but valuing winning over the game is not the goal.** This is an especially important message in order to keep things fun and inclusive for family members of all ages.

☐ **Mix it up!** Board or card games, frisbee, scavenger hunts, puzzles, dance parties – if it gets the family playing together and having a blast, well...mission accomplished!

A few classics (and future classics) to add to your repertoire: Jenga, Pictionary, Scattergories, Operation, Monopoly, Go Fish!,

Apples to Apples, Uno, Balderdash, Simon Says, Scrabble, Twister...
What are your favorites?

Helpful hint: No need to lighten your wallet unnecessarily. In addition to absolutely free options (Hide and Seek or Charades, for instance), check the shelves at local thrift stores for cheap deals on board games, scour garage sales, or start a game library for trading with friends and family.

## AMPLIFY YOUR EFFORTS.

Keep the positive vibes rolling...

☐ **Commit to making game night a weekly (or every-other-week) event.**

☐ **Host an expanded game night by inviting another family to join in.**

---

# RESOURCES:

Ankowski A, Ankowski A: *Bringing back family game night*, 2015. Available at: http://www.pbs.org/parents/expert-tips-advice/2015/07/bringing-back-family-game-night/.

Efe B: *20 Family game night ideas*, 2018. Available at: www.playtivities.com/20-family-game-night-ideas/.

Harac L: *The benefits of family game time*. Available at: http://www.schoolfamily.com/school-family-articles/article/10895-the-benefits-of-family-game-time.

Markham L: *The family that plays together*, 2021. Available at: https://www.mkewithkids.com/post/family-that-plays-together-stays-together

Merrill S: *20 ideas for a family fun night*. Available at: https://www.imom.com/20-ideas-for-a-family-fun-night/

# NOTES:

# 19

## KEEP IT *Routine*

"Some nights at our house are like a blissful depiction of a TV family. A lot of nights at least one kid's big feelings get the best of them and the emotions come out through tears, yelling or bouncing off the walls. While the melodrama of our life looks different every night, we try to keep one thing consistent: our bedtime routine. For our family it includes one-on-one time with each of my kids. For my 6-year-old, it's a little extra snuggle time. For my 9-year-old, it's a chance to ask questions about what she heard the older kids talking about on the playground. The whole process doesn't have to be pretty or perfect, because let's face it, there's not a lot about parenting that is. It just has to be predictable and planful."

Days that quietly end with the kids snuggling on the sofa – jammies on, teeth brushed, ready to pop contentedly into bed – well, they feel like one in a million. Or maybe two in 365. At any rate, they're rare.

For many of us, evenings are typically more chaotic than calm. Homework is challenging. Somebody lost the leggings that they *have to* wear to school tomorrow. Your schedule for tomorrow just changed. The entire vibe is less than blissful.

Lucky for us, generations of previous parents toiled to crack the code on this daily struggle and came up with a game-changing tool: routines.

While words like "structure" and "routine" may cause some adults to break out in a rebellious sweat, routines are a balm for kids whose entire lives are about constant change over which they have very little control. Routines give them something they can count on, provide security, and help build self-discipline.

Transitioning from a normal day's activities to settling down is a challenge for many—which makes bedtime routines especially important. For some, bedtime is when kids finally slow down enough to start worrying about how problems from today might carry over into tomorrow. It's a lot for a kid or even a teen to process. Building consistent routines early can help diminish worries down the road.

## PREDICTABILITY, ALL DAY LONG.

Strict routines are more important for some kids, and some adults, than others. You know what kind of people you are, so operate in a way that works for your family and preserves everybody's sense of peace. In most cases, aim for 'predictable' versus 'regimented' for the best results.

Try breaking your day into segments: morning, after school, mealtime, bedtime, etc. A sample approach to a typical school day might look like this:

☐ **Morning.** Wake up the kids up on a positive note. Trilling out "Good morning, sunshine!" is a totally acceptable substitute for an alarm clock and will most certainly lodge in their brains to be passed on to the next generation. Make sure they eat breakfast and then send them off to school with a kiss, hug or "Have a fantastic day!" It sets a tone of positivity and possibility.

☐ **After School.** If your children come home directly after school, have some healthy snacks available and spend a few minutes chatting about their day. When you ask about what happened at school, you're might to get a "Nothing" in response – totally unsatisfying, but ask anyway. Allow them some space to relax before they tackle homework.

*Important note: If at all possible, kids up through the middle school years should come home to a responsible adult or adolescent as opposed to an empty home. Teens should check in with a parent when they arrive home as well – even if it is by phone.*

☐ **Dinner Time.** Getting everybody to sit down together every night can be hard when you consider parental work schedules and after school activities for the kids. If you can't do it every night, at least try for a few nights a week where you all sit down together and talk with all electronic devices off or put away (see Chapter 29). And while you're at it, enlist the kids to help set the table or prepare the meal. Attempt to keep dinner at a somewhat consistent time most evenings.

☐ **Bedtime.** Wind down by enforcing a "no screens" deadline – at least 45 minutes before bed – to help signal to kids' brains and bodies that it is time to prepare for sleep. Do your best to stick to a pre-determined bedtime hour. To make the next morning easier, have the kids select what clothing they want to wear, what things they need to take with them, and get everything ready to go. Have them, or help them, brush their teeth, bathe, and put on their pajamas. Then read the little ones a story or two before tucking them into bed. Make it a priority to spend some one-on-one time with each child.

When creating a new family routine, ask the kids for their input if appropriate. Then, be sure to explain the new plan so everybody knows what to expect. Put it in writing if that helps, and be patient as you work out the kinks while the family adjusts.

## AMPLIFY YOUR EFFORTS.

Kids aren't the only ones who benefit from routines. Big people need structure, too! Be sure to carve out regular "parent nights" and workout times – and stick to them. Map out your day the night before to be sure you get things done and are moving toward your own personal goals. This can also help make for a less-frazzled morning.

And, after you've successfully put the kids to bed at a *reasonable* time, try to put up your feet, relax and renew yourself. It all starts again in the morning!

## RESOURCES:

Aha! Parenting.com: *Why kids need routines.* 2019. Available at: www. ahaparenting.com/parenting-tools/family-life/structure-routines.

Head Start/ECLKS: The importance of schedules and routines. 2020. Available at: https://eclkc.ohs.acf.hhs.gov/about-us/article/ importance-schedules-routines

KidsRKids: *Child won't follow a routine or schedule? Try these tips.* 2021. Available at: https://kidsrkids.com/avalon-park/2021/10/08/ child-wont-follow-a-routine-try-these-tips/

# NOTES:

# 20
## *Get* A MOVE ON

"Getting my kids up off the couch or off their cell phones and moving is a struggle – and adding in a pandemic and schooling from home didn't help. So, I try to inject exercise in fun ways: walking them to a friend's house or riding our bikes to the grocery store. Sometimes I'll even challenge them to a jumping jacks or push-ups contest. It actually gets everybody both sweating and giggling!"

The joys of huffing, puffing and breaking a good old-fashioned sweat are *way* underrated. Sure, families who sweat together log more showers and have more robust stinky sock piles than others, but ohhhh the rewards! Even just a few minutes of exercise a day is great for you, it's great for your kids, and it's doubly great when you do it together.

A brief refresher on a few fantastic things regular exercise can do for kids (and you!):

- Build strong muscles and bones
- Help keep a healthy weight
- Promote a more positive outlook and reduce the risk for depression
- Increase concentration and improve test scores
- Build self-esteem
- Lower stress

According to the US Department of Health and Human Services, children between the ages of six and 17 years should be logging 60 minutes a day of physical activity. Younger kids should be given multiple opportunities for physical play throughout the day. But it doesn't have to be in one, hour-long chunk! Even short bursts of activity add up. And you don't really have to work up a sweat to have exercise be healthy, although sweating is a good sign the workout was vigorous.

Plenty of children get the exercise they need through organized team sports, but those aren't for everyone. And even those kids may need a gentle push to keep moving and developing habits that will serve them well into adulthood. Your challenge: come up with ways to keep things fun, interesting and somewhat sweat-inducing!

## 1-2-3-ACTIVATE!

Grown-ups, lace up your running shoes or hiking boots, ice skates, flippers, whatever. Setting an example of being physically active for – and with – your kids can help lead them toward the mindset that an active lifestyle rocks! In some households, the phrase "let's get some exercise" is met with eye rolls and moans. If you make activities fun, kids might not realize what they're doing is actually viewed by some as a workout. Some ideas to get everyone up and at 'em:

- ☐ **Make it a dance party!** It's always a great day to get your groove on – and it doesn't even require going outside. Crank up the tunes and start moving. It's infectious – truly.

- ☐ **Cha cha through your chores.** Bump things up a notch. Stick a dust rag in one kid's hand and a vacuum cleaner in the other's and make it a dance/work party.

- ☐ **Take a hike.** Locate a park or nature trail – even an interesting nearby neighborhood – and go. Bring a few healthy snacks and water along to make it feel like an adventure – and appreciate the plants, animals, and scenery. Set your sights on a half or full-day hike and work towards that goal.

- [ ] **Sign up for a walk or run for charity.** Do it together. Many events also offer shorter races just for kids.

- [ ] **Bike, don't drive.** Need a few things from the store? If you can, try walking or cycling there and back instead of automatically hopping in the car.

- [ ] **Have a field day.** Invite some friends and turn your yard or a nearby park into a mini-Olympic stadium. Fun but simple activities could include badminton or volleyball, frisbee golf, lots of relays or a long jump competition. Get creative!

- [ ] **Run through the sprinkler.** Guaranteed to induce squeals and laughter.

Kids feeling restless? Have them do jumping jacks. Siblings growing grouchy? Prescribe a family hike. Walk the dog. Rake leaves, then jump in them. Play tag. Take the stairs. Wash the car by hand. Challenge yourself to park in the hinterlands of the mall parking lot without it ruining your mood! Every day provides endless opportunities to simply move. Look for them.

## AMPLIFY YOUR EFFORTS.

Focus on safety and positivity to ensure every kid is both physically protected and feels included in any activity. Not everyone is born to be a star athlete, but nearly everyone can participate at some level.

- [ ] Be sure kids use proper gear (helmets, shoes, etc.) when needed, and model the same. And be present! Especially around water or other high-risk activities, your attention and supervision are critical.

- [ ] Prioritize swim lessons for your children and teach them to always ask you if they can go in or near the water. Drowning is a leading cause of death for children, according to the American Red Cross.

☐ Think twice before signing your kids up for one-on-one coaching (see Chapter 32 for more on this topic). Group activities are safer and more fun.

## RESOURCES:

Gilmore, M. *Why dancing round your living room should be a family affair.* 2016. Available at: www.express.co.uk/life-style/life/648201/Why-dancing-living-room-should-family-affair.

Great Ormond Street Hospital for Children: *Exercise for children and young people,* 2013. Available at: http://www.gosh.nhs.uk/medical-information/general-health-advice/leading-active-lifestyle/exercise-children-and-young-people.

Mayo Clinic: *How much exercise a day do children need?* 2019. Available at: www.mayoclinic.org/healthy-lifestyle/fitness/expert-answers/kids-and-exercise/faq-20058336.

Watts C: *Move more not less. Our kids are our future: Understanding exercise for kids.* Available at: https://www.linkedin.com/pulse/move-more-less-our-kids-future-understanding-exercise-chris-watts

# NOTES:

# 21
## PLANT A *Garden*

"Some of my earliest memories are of helping my mom in her vegetable garden—laying a ruler along the ground to plant seeds at the correct width, thinning carrots to the right spacing, digging potatoes with my bare hands. There is nothing quite like the unforgettable taste of a carrot, freshly pulled from the ground, that still has a nice little coating of dirt on it. As an adult with a busy life and career, I rediscovered the meditative and rewarding act of gardening because of children—specifically, working with volunteers helping preschoolers explore the world of gardening with wonder and fresh eyes. It's not just about the end result of the harvest, but planning, planting, watching, nurturing, tasting, and letting go of perfect control to witness something miraculous."

Stroll through a garden in the full bloom of summer and just *try* to resist indulging in the savory 'pop' of a cherry tomato, the sweet bliss of a perfectly ripened raspberry, or a freshly cut bouquet of cheerful daisies. The colors! The smells! The flavors! The bounty!

A garden is a little slice of awesome in our otherwise fast-paced, electronics-fueled world. It's a place to get your hands dirty, be creative, and – if you're dedicated – even save some cash on groceries.

So, what's in it for kids? Plenty. For starters, kids are notorious vegetable resistors. Might they be more likely to give carrots or

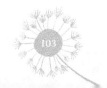

cucumbers a go if they grow the goods themselves? It's certainly food for thought. But there are many more positives to tending a family garden than healthier eating preferences.

Here's what else digging and planting a garden can cultivate in kids:

- **Reduced stress.** Many adults garden in order to slow down, enjoy the many rewards of working the earth, and clear the mind of intrusive thoughts and concerns. Why would it be any different for kids?
- **A love of science and math.** Planning a garden can nurture children's analytical and research abilities. Detail-loving kids can turn the process into a science experiment by researching and implementing what to plant, where to plant it, the best time of year for growing different crops, how water and soil impact success, etc.
- **An opportunity for fresh air and exercise.** Digging + raking = weight training + cardio!
- **Better moods and more confidence.** It's empowering for kids to plant seeds, water them, and watch them blossom. It encourages taking responsibility and has an exciting payoff. And it's especially rewarding for children to know they're contributing to the family by helping grow food you eat together.

## SOW WHAT?

According to experts, carrots, potatoes, cherry tomatoes, radishes, sugar snap peas, and pumpkins are among the easiest and hardiest crops for the garden. And don't forget flowers! Sunflowers and nasturtiums are favorites.

To get started, decide where you're able to plant. You don't need a large backyard – or any backyard at all. Many a tomato and lettuce head have been harvested from containers on apartment balconies. Or maybe your area has a community garden where you can plant. Aim for good light and quality soil.

From there: Invest in a few basic gardening tools.

☐ Supervise your child, but let them do most of the heavy lifting in getting things established. Step in when necessary to help out. The goal here is success.

☐ Let them do the harvesting and preparing of food as age allows.

## AMPLIFY YOUR EFFORTS.

☐ **Do some healthy bragging.** Make sure family members and others know about your child's efforts and success. It will drive home that their work truly matters.

☐ **Snap lots of pictures to document progress.**

☐ **Plan a neighborhood or extended family feast with the bounty of the garden and celebrate!**

☐ **Encourage your child to share the harvest with neighbors, or better yet, see if a local food pantry could use your fresh produce.** Search www.ampleharvest.org for one near you.

---

# RESOURCES:

Schmurak S: *Get your kids in the garden.* 2016. Eartheasy. Available at: https://learn.eartheasy.com/articles/get-your-kids-in-the-garden/

Flavin B: *Gardening for kids: 7 reasons planting seeds enriches their lives,* 2016. Available at: www.rasmussen.edu/degrees/education/blog/gardening-for-kids-benefits/.

Grant B: *Garden activities for teens: how to garden with teenagers.* Available at: https://www.gardeningknowhow.com/special/children/gardening-with-teenagers.htm

kidsgardening.org: www.kidsgardening.org website. (Subscription).

## NOTES:

# 22
# Dampen THE DECIBELS

"I'm one of four siblings, so growing up in our house was never very quiet. But now that we're all married and have children of our own, the noise level at our family gatherings has gone from 'I think this is normal,' to 'I hope the neighbors don't complain.' We now have a wild mix of enthusiastic voices, laughter, screaming (are they playing or are they fighting?) and the sound of little feet tearing through the house and slamming doors. I admit, sometimes the volume reaches headache-inducing heights. However, spending time as a family is just plain worth it. And while we are all still figuring out this parenting thing together, I suppose if the kids are laughing (yes, and sometimes screaming), we must be doing something right."

Let's just get the math on this out of the way first thing. The equation goes like this:

One kid + more kids = LOTS of noise.

To add to that, the addition of even one more child to a group automatically raises the overall decibel level by an unfathomable multiple. Groups of kids seem to love nothing more than to scream and yell and pretty much raise the roof right off the house.

*And maybe you're finding it overwhelming.* For some of us, loud

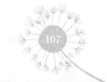

noise is a source of tremendous stress. When it comes to kids and noise and chaos, what's tolerable depends a lot on your personality, current mood, and past life experiences. For some people, loud, continuous crying or screaming provokes feelings of frustration and even anger. (Note: A single wailing newborn or tantrum-y toddler can have the same impact, and then some. For more on how to deal with that particular source of noise, please see Chapter 40, Keep Your Cool).

In all honestly, who *doesn't* start losing their patience sometimes when chaos seems to be breaking loose around us? As adults and parents, it's our job to find ways to cope, whether that means providing new (and hopefully, quieter) distractions, firmly setting expectations or changing the vibe within the household.

## LISTEN UP.

Step number one: identify and assess the source of the noise and upheaval that is making you feel a little stressed. Are the kids having a truly good time – giggling and playing games or are things leaning more in the direction of a conflict that requires immediate adult intervention? In other words, separate "good noise" from "bad noise" and take a moment to plan your reaction accordingly.

Now, you can decide which tactic is going to work best in the moment:

☐ **Turn down the noise where you can.** Assess whether other factors are contributing to your angst. Small annoyances like the TV, music, washing machine, vacuum cleaner or your neighbor's lawnmower could be making things worse. See if there is anything you can change right now to lower the noise level – and hopefully, your stress level.

☐ **Allot a controlled amount of time (maybe 2-3 minutes) for the kids to be as loud as they want.** This might involve pots and pans and stomping and screaming, but when the three minutes are up? That's it.

☐ **If you can, get some exercise to clear your head, or add a few minutes of meditation to your day.**

☐ **Don't YELL.** *Whisper* (i.e., be the change you want to see in your household). Child behavior experts support whispering or lowering your voice to kids as an antidote to yelling, to encourage them to listen, and to calm them.

☐ **Remind the kids there's a time and a place for antics.** Acknowledge that it's not acceptable for children to be off-the-hook loud or disruptive in, say, a restaurant, store, or church. Gently remind them to use their "inside voices," or maybe they need to just take the noise outdoors.

☐ **Consider earplugs.** With tiny kids, you certainly need to be alert to what they're up to at all times. As they get older, you have a bit more flexibility. As long as you are not totally shut out from what's happening in your household, a little muffling can be a great thing!

## AMPLIFY YOUR EFFORTS.

"Amplify" may be the last thing you want to hear, but this is important: if you find your efforts to quiet your children are failing, or that you are having difficulty coping with your own frustration levels, seek the help of a qualified parenting expert or therapist to get to the bottom of the issue and help restore a sense of calm and control.

## RESOURCES:

Andrews J: *Efforts to quiet a noisy family starts with quieter parents,* 2020. Available at: https://www.producer.com/farmliving/efforts-to-quiet-a-noisy-family-starts-with-quieter-parents/

Knost LR: *The incredible power of the whisper,* 2013. Available at: https://www.littleheartsbooks.com/2013/07/03/the-incredible-power-of-the-whisper/.

Markham L: *Your 10-point plan to stop yelling,* 2018. Available at: https://www.ahaparenting.com/read/Plan-to-Stop-Yelling

Sturiale J: *Stop yelling at your kids.* Available at: www.webmd.com/parenting/features/stop-yelling-at-your-kids#1.

---

# NOTES:

# 23
## LET THEM *Play*

> "In my experience raising children, I found unstructured play time not only valuable for my kids, but incredibly nurturing and energizing for myself. Time spent building forts, exploring, slaying dragons, and creating Lego worlds gave me a glorious window into the minds of my children and their interests while also allowing me time to relax, de-stress and act a little bit like a kid myself."

Here we go, adding *one more thing* to your to-do list. But this one's fun, free and doesn't require a carpool, we promise. Open your calendar and jot this down somewhere between 'school,' 'work' and 'chores': P-L-A-Y. That's right, play. We're talking climbing trees, digging in the dirt, splashing in the pool, running through the yard, playing "pretend," uninhibited kind of play.

Somewhere in our rush to cram kids' schedules with academics, sports, piano lessons, art classes, jobs and other things that monopolize their time and ours, we're robbing them of the opportunity to simply play. Most of us adults apparently didn't get enough of it either. Playtime has been on the decline since 1955! So, unless you're a big exception to the rule, your kids could probably use one less math worksheet and a few more minutes of freedom. Because as far as child development goes, playing is pretty serious business.

Experts point out that unstructured play:

**Builds kids' brains and bodies.** All that running around and imaginative time flings the doors wide open to possibility. Kids are free to discover what truly interests them. They also learn skills such as negotiation, collaboration, empathy, problem-solving and decision-making – on their own terms.

**Strengthens the parent-child bond.** Sure it does! Playing together lets your kids see your fun-loving side and provides time to just *be* together. Plus, it feels good to surrender to a game of tag, pitch in to play store or work on a puzzle.

**Helps with social relationships.** Playing together bonds kids with shared memories, while building skills centered around inter-action, sharing, and cooperation.

**Teaches them independence and creativity.** Having time to operate outside the confines of a classroom or other structured setting enables children to build the skills they need to take charge of their own lives.

**Encourages joy.** Play is an antidote to fear and stress – a magic elixir that transforms kids into royalty or superheroes, scientists or astronauts, ready to take on their own little corner of the world. Play gives kids opportunities to discover their true passions.

## READY. SET. PLAY!

The beauty of setting kids free to play is that there are no rules. Feel free to make suggestions and participate, especially with small children, but for the most part, let them be the boss!

Your end of the deal?

☐ **Supervise, and ensure play areas are safe.**

☐ **As a playmate to younger kids, follow their lead.** Ask "What do *you* want to play?"

☐ **Expect to repeat activities as they develop skills.** You might, for instance, find yourself being served 27 pretend cups of tea as the lone guest of an elaborate tea party. Just go with it.

☐ **Brainstorm ways you can add an element of play to everyday activities**. Make up silly songs or stories in the car as you run errands, or turn household chores into a game by having kids dress up in their favorite costume and fold laundry or dust the furniture in character.

☐ **Laugh as much as possible**!

## AMPLIFY YOUR EFFORTS.

Don't think for one minute that play is only for kids. We need to laugh and let loose as much as they do. So dance, climb a tree, go ice skating or bowling, or color in a coloring book. Whatever you choose – embrace it and have the most fun possible.

**Try this.** Grab some sheets or blankets from the linen closet and have the kids help drape them over a table, chairs or other furniture to create a cool hideout. *Maybe* they'll come out for dinner!

---

# RESOURCES:

Bongiorno L: *10 things every parent should know about play.* National Association for the Education of Young Children. Available at: https://www.naeyc.org/our-work/families/10-things-every-parent-play

Hill D: *For Black children, play can be transformative,* 2021. Available at: https://greatergood.berkeley.edu/article/item/for_black_children_play_can_be_transformative

Milteer R & Ginsburg K: The importance of play in promoting healthy child development and maintaining strong parent-child bond: Focus on children in poverty. 2012. Available at: https://publications.aap.org/pediatrics/article/129/1/e204/31545/The-Importance-of-Play-in-Promoting-Child?autologincheck=redirect

# NOTES:

# 24

# *Be* SPONTANEOUS (ONCE IN A WHILE)

"It's so important to be spontaneous that you should start doing these 14 things... Nope! That's not how this one works, though spontaneity does require effort. On the other side of the planned and scheduled life are genuine treasures – 'for real' moments with friends, family, animals, strangers – all reminders of the lovely moments life has to offer."

So you're a scheduler. The kind of planner who feels a chill run down your spine when you imagine having to deviate from your well-oiled nap/meals/school/bath/bedtime routine. We get it. For some of us, it can feel as if all that's holding the world together is a little masking tape, chewing gum and an airtight schedule.

But, what if...? What if tonight, bedtime was at 8:30 instead of 7:30, or you served McNuggets two nights in a row, or allowed nap time to take place *during a car ride*? Would it all fall apart? We're here to say that it just might not.

Yes, kids need routines. But your mission, should you choose to accept it, is to – occasionally – let a few things go. Let the dinner dishes soak a bit longer and instead spend some time building a pillow fort, step outside to enjoy a lovely sunset, or hustle out the door to catch a free lecture at a local museum.

We call this phenomenon *spontaneity,* and for the Type A

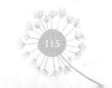

planners and rule followers out there, surrendering to a bit of it once in a while can rock your world – in some very rewarding ways.

Structure and schedules and goals and consistency help kids evolve into strong, resilient adults. But encouraging them to be spontaneous helps them be *human*. Unstructured time feeds the soul, stokes the fire of personality and keeps us all feeling young.

Encouraging spontaneity in your kids also helps build:

- Problem solving skills
- Comfort with ambiguity (No road map? No problem!)
- The ability to navigate change
- Confidence
- Creativity and imagination

So let loose. There is something freeing about letting go of expectations – embracing the fact that plans often go sideways anyway – and instead improvising new, different, even better plans on-the-fly.

## DECONSTRUCT YOUR STRUCTURE.

Most kids seem naturally geared for unplanned adventures. Among adults, some seem to have inherited a spontaneity "gene," while others will only leave their neighborhood after 6 p.m. if the house is on fire. If you're in the first camp, the idea of needing instructions on how to fly by the seat of your pants probably sounds ridiculous. But for others, here we are with some step-by-step instructions for how to get your impulse on.

☐ Step 1. **Clear some space in your calendar by saying goodbye to something.** Do the kids need to be scheduled from dawn to dusk seven days a week, or might one or two things be dropped to allow everybody a chance to chill out and do what sounds fun in the moment?

☐ Step 2. **Know that dinner and bedtime routines are important, but they're not *everything*.** Given the right set of circumstances, it might be worth staying up late to work together on an ambitious Halloween costume, try one more science experiment before school the next day, or catch the last showing of a film. You might even bond more!

☐ Step 3. **Brace for spur-of-the-moment inspiration.** It's okay to occasionally drop weekend plans in favor of an impromptu trip, an afternoon spent acting like tourists in your hometown, or a fully unstructured day of jumping in mud puddles, making pizza from scratch, or assembling the most complicated puzzle ever.

☐ Step 4. **Turn the unexpected into something worth remembering.** Flight cancelled? Explore the airport, check out the displays reflecting local pride, watch the tarmac activities, or see if other travelers are game for some small talk about where they're traveling. The goal here is, when plans change due to circumstances beyond your control, embrace it.

## AMPLIFY YOUR EFFORTS.

Still having a hard time letting loose? Try this odd – but oddly logical – suggestion: *Plan some spontaneity.* Extreme circumstances call for extreme measures.

Clear your schedule this Saturday and just hang out. Play some games, watch a family movie, go for a nature walk, bake cookies. Do whatever sounds fun or rewarding and see how you feel at the end of the day. Invigorated and inspired, we hope.

And, *ssshhhh.* Don't tell the kids you actually planned an event-free day. They'll think you're all kinds of fun.

# RESOURCES:

Armstrong T: Book review of Elkind D: The power of play: how spontaneous, imaginative activities lead to happier, healthier children, *J Play* 1(1):126-128, 2008. Available at: www. journalofplay.org/issues/1/1/book-review/power-play-how-spontaneous-imaginative-activities-lead-happier-healthier. (Table of contents for multiple play articles)/

Burnett C: *Responding to children's spontaneous experimentation*, 2019. Available at: www. childhood101.com/responding-to-childrens-spontaneous-experimentation/.

Hewes J: Seeking balance in motion: The role of spontaneous free play in promoting social and emotional health in early childhood care and education, *Children* 1(3):280-301, 2014, Available at: www. ncbi.nlm.nih.gov/pmc/articles/PMC4928743/.

Seltzer L: *The wisdom of spontaneity (part 2): are you spontaneous or impulsive?...and why you should care*, 2009. Available at: https://www.psychologytoday.com/us/blog/evolution-the-self/200904/the-wisdom-spontaneity-part-2/

# NOTES:

# 25

# Laugh. A LOT.

> "The sound of my toddler's laughter is just about the best sound I have ever heard. Nothing brings me into the moment more than hearing those giggles. It's magical."

**M**oments of genuine, uncontrollable, make-your-eyes-water sort of laughter are like an instant workout for your soul. One second you'll be sitting there having an ordinary sort of day and a few minutes later, your abs have gotten a workout, your cheeks are throbbing and you're recovering from that hilarious snorting sound you made.

It's a choice, really. We can journey through life wringing our hands and taking everything so... very... seriously. Or we can work to spot the humor. Even in the dark moments. Even in hard situations. Even when every other bone in our body says *Ugh*, we've still got a funny bone, right?

Aside from feeling oh-so-amazing, laughter and a healthy sense of humor actually works behind the scenes to accomplish some pretty cool things. It can:

- Help relieve stress (all part of that 'feeling amazing' sensation)
- Get your internal organs moving (increasing oxygen intake and circulation, benefiting your heart, lungs and muscles and releasing those magical endorphins)

- Boost the immune system and help relieve pain
- Put you in a better mood – and potentially even help increase life satisfaction

For children, the benefits are even greater. Laughter and a sense of humor play a role in building self-esteem and resilience, encouraging creative thinking and problem-solving skills, seeing things from new perspectives and learning not to take themselves too seriously. Kids learn best when they are playing and having fun, so by all means, inject every bit of fun and laughter into all your shared experiences as you possibly can.

## PUMP UP THE FUNNY.

Sometimes, laughter can truly be the best medicine – particularly in situations where there is no official medicine or easy solution that can tidily fix things up. The ability to reframe a situation into something that looks different, more hopeful, and perhaps even humorous, is a powerful skill to take into adulthood. Fortunately, finding humor is a skill that can be taught.

How?

☐ **Tell corny jokes.** "Knock, knock. *Who's there?* Closure. *Closure who?* Closure mouth while you're chewing!" Now there's a way to teach your kids manners while keeping it light. Try to introduce appropriate jokes and humor in place of what might be viewed as 'boring old parent' behavior.

☐ **Be silly and laugh along with them.** It's a great way to relate to and bond with your kids. But also, know where to draw the line. While humor is an incredible tool, not everything is funny and not everybody will appreciate your (or your kids') particular brand of humor. Be mindful and respectful. Laugh *with* people, not *at* them.

☐ **Share funny things that happen in your day.** Recounting things that happen to you in a good-natured, entertaining way can encourage the same ability in your children.

☐ **Read funny stories and watch fun family movies together.**

☐ **Help your kids see the bright side of things,** and keep life events in perspective. The example you set is their guide.

☐ **Keep it positive.** The point of good humor is never to tear others down. Discourage off-color jokes or humor that is at the expense of another.

☐ **Don't take yourself too seriously,** and encourage your children not to either. People who can more readily roll with challenges and find humor in difficult circumstances are likely to find themselves both healthier and happier.

## AMPLIFY YOUR EFFORTS.

Feeling serious about this funny business? Double your efforts by having a family joke night, where kids and parents are tasked with sharing a few jokes.

Or, analyze what could be seen as an unfortunate or unfunny situation (the car breaking down on family vacation, a disagreement with someone, a series of annoying events throughout the day) and deliberately look for the humor that might be hiding there. Discuss it together and challenge each other to go out into the world with a 'glass half full' mentality, ready to embrace the humor in each day.

---

## RESOURCES:

All Pro Dad: *10 ways to teach your child to be funny.* Available at: www. allprodad.com/10-ways-to-teach-your-children-to-be-funny/.

Gavin M: *Encouraging your child's sense of humor,* 2015. Available at: https://kidshealth.org/en/parents/child-humor.html

Live Life With Your Kids: *Laugh with your family,* n.d. Available at: https://www.livelifewithyourkids.com/2016/07/laugh-family/

Mayo Clinic Staff: *Stress relief from laughter? It's no joke.* April 5, 2019. Available at: www.mayoclinic.org/healthy-lifestyle/stress-management/in-depth/stress-relief/art-20044456.

Pool C, Miller SA, Church EB: *Ages & Stages: Don't forget to laugh! The importance of humor.* Available at: www.scholastic.com/teachers/articles/teaching-content/ages-stages-dont-forget-laugh-importance-humor/.

Vondruska B: *Stop laughing at your kids,* 2019. Available at: https://www.thekindofparentyouare.com/articles/stop-laughing

---

# NOTES:

# 26
## GET *Outdoors!*

"When my brother was about eight years old, he and his buddies conducted a 'science experiment' where they tied some helium balloons together, attached a questionnaire that they had carefully written and stuffed into a plastic bag to keep it dry, then launched their aircraft. (Sure, it got stuck in the trees a few times, but eventually they figured it out.) Several months later, they got a letter back with their questionnaire completed. The boys were elated! The balloon had sailed all the way across Lake Michigan from Illinois to Michigan where it ended up in a field. Their work paid off, while at the same time they had a blast being outside, using their minds and 'experimenting' with nature."

You know that powerful sense of "Wow!" that comes when you've caught a spectacular sunset, or observed a firefly *lighting up*, or – if you're lucky enough – witnessed an eclipse? Yeah, those experiences that nature hands out as generously as free candy are hard to come by when you're stuck inside all day.

Mother Nature is a pretty amazing thing. Whether it's experienced on a dramatic scale – like a trip to the Grand Canyon – or more accessible from the convenience of your neighborhood, nature has the power to soothe and heal.

More than half of the world's population lives in cities or urban environments – a number that is expected to grow to 70% over the next few decades. As this urbanization has increased, so too has the rate of mental disorders, including depression. Coincidence? We think not, say researchers at Stanford. They urge us – kids and adults alike – to take regular breathers from buildings, vehicles, excessive noise and crowds and spend some time in more open, natural spaces.

Getting away from the urban rush and acquainted with nature can:

- Lower stress levels
- Improve symptoms of anxiety and depression
- Improve cognition for kids challenged by attention deficits
- Make us more positive and generous humans (all that awe and gratitude we mentioned earlier)
- Spark curiosity and creativity
- Help with memory
- Inspire a love of the natural sciences
- Get kids off the couch, away from their screens and moving!

Promoting the value and beauty of nature is also bound to spark love and appreciation for the Earth in younger generations. Hearing a 4-year-old look at an oily puddle after a rain shower and saying "Oh, a rainbow melted!" is the sort of thing that can make your day – a benefit that is more critical now than ever.

## IT'S IN THEIR NATURE.

You don't have to plan an emergency trip to Yellowstone Park or adopt a polar bear in order to introduce your kids to the outdoors. (Do, however, take advantage of travel opportunities when you can. Feel free to leave the polar bears in the arctic).

Here's what you *can* do, maybe even today:

☐ **Start simple. Get the kids out in the yard to play a game, or just to lie on the grass and look for cloud shapes in the sky.** Extra credit if you decide to pitch a tent and stage a backyard campout.

☐ **Find a park, grab your kids and go.** There are likely two or three within reasonable distance of your home. Got a state or national park nearby? Lucky you!

☐ **Take a hike.** Even big cities usually have walking or hiking trails nearby that can feel like a genuine urban escape. Turn it into a true nature hike by challenging the kids to spot birds and animals, or collect leaves to identify later.

☐ **Go fishing.** Google "kids fishing near me" to find kid-friendly fishing holes.

☐ **Place a birdhouse in your yard, or plant flowers that attract bumblebees and other insects.** Talk about the creatures that visit your yard.

☐ **Model a sense of wonder** about what you discover together in nature.

☐ **Wherever you are, stop and smell the flowers.** Literally.

## AMPLIFY YOUR EFFORTS.

As your little ones evolve into teens, it can become harder to coax them away from their screens and their friends for outdoor (or indoor) family time. Which presents a new challenge for you to be creative.

Even the most reluctant teens might be convinced to convene with nature if it includes ziplining or a ropes course. Others may be enticed by rock climbing, a rafting or kayaking day, a camping weekend or a wilderness camp (without parents!) Got a creative soul in your brood? Encourage them to bring along a musical instrument, painting supplies, camera or a journal to capture their observations in a way that inspires them.

Many high schools require students to complete volunteer hours in order to meet graduation requirements. Help your child find an outdoor opportunity – such as a local park cleanup or invasive plant removal project – where they can get their hands dirty while also doing a good deed. And many teens are now responding to the climate change challenges. They want to do things to clean up the environment and make it healthier for the future.

Nature is for everyone, yet only 9% of the 144.4 million Americans who participated in outdoor recreation in 2016 were Black due to historic issues related to culture, economics and fears surrounding safety. All of us – regardless of racial or ethnic background – can find power, confidence and healing in natural spaces. If you feel reluctant to take those first steps into exploring outdoor spaces, know that there are organizations that promote and guide Black youth and families in outdoor programs, even on trips to national and state parks. You can find them online for your area.

It's nature for the win!

---

# RESOURCES:

Comeriato HL: *Nature gap: Outdoor recreation isn't just for white people. Invite Black youth outside*, USA Today, 2020. Available at: https://www.usatoday.com/story/opinion/voices/2020/10/29/nature-environment-race-black-recreation-report-for-america/6054520002/

Cohen D: *Why kids need to spend time in nature*, 2021. Childmind Institute. Available at: https://www.childmind.org/article/why-kids-need-to-spend-time-in-nature/

Louv R: Leave no child inside: the remedy for environmental despair is as close as the front door. *Sierra Magazine*, July/August 2006. Available at: https://vault.sierraclub.org/sierra/200607/child.asp

One Tough Job: *100 books about getting outside*, 2021. Available at: http://www.onetoughjob.org/articles/nature-exploration-books-601-700

Parent.co. *Why time outdoors can increase kids' ability to focus,* 2021. Available at: https:www.parent.com/blogs/conversations/ why-time-outdoors-can-increase-kids-ability-to-focus

---

NOTES:

# 27

# TO HAVE, TO HOLD AND TO *Blend*

"When I was in high school, my mom met her second husband, a fabulous man with three young children. The 'little kids' lived with us half of the year, which was a big adjustment for all of us. My brother, sister, and I had always been a tight team of three. Now we were taking on the role of older siblings and sharing the time and attention of our mom. Slowly and steadily, this new family framework took shape. There was no magic moment of perfect harmony; time created connections and our parents continually worked on positive family dynamics. Were there challenges? Absolutely! Did we fight? Of course! Were there days we wished it would go back to the way it was? Sometimes. Would I change the story? No way. Today, we are all close – a family unit that looks out for each other and shares a special kind of family connection."

Mike and Carol Brady made it look SO easy on their hit 1970s TV show *The Brady Bunch*. Six zany kids, a jovial housekeeper, antics galore – and no problem that couldn't be resolved in 30 minutes, including commercials. And the clincher, of course, was that theirs was a *blended* family that began, as most do, with the one day when the lady met this fellow.

Stepparents – and future stepparents – take heed: The Bradys set the bar high. Entering into a new life that combines children,

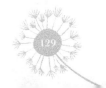

multiple parents plus extended families, ongoing family conflicts, hectic schedules and divergent personalities can be rough going.

Your toddler stepdaughter may not be quite so "charming" once you're living together on a full-time basis. Your teenage son could have major problems with being disciplined by somebody who's "not my dad." New siblings have big adjustments to face, and there's the ever-evolving potential minefield of ex-partner dynamics. None of this stuff is easy.

On the flip side, putting in the work to build a family with new traditions and an expanded network of people who are on your – and your kids' – team can be one of life's greatest joys and one of the most love-filled things you might ever give your children.

Note: Up to now we've talked about ways to build the stability and strength of your existing family. But sometimes new families are created when adults with children come together as a blended family. If that situation represents your family, we are here with a few tips for you.

## THIS GROUP MUST SOMEHOW FORM A FAMILY.

We're taking this Brady Bunch theme all the way to the end zone. Combining families means forging ahead, fully committed. At the same time, harmony and understanding can't be forced.

Excitement, uncertainty, sadness, anger, jealousy. Your kids are guaranteed to have plenty of feelings about this new family you're forming. Children under age 10 or so are likely to adjust more quickly than pre-teens and teens, who are apt to balk at accepting discipline from a new person.

Other factors that will impact your kids' adjustment timetable include things like how long it has been since their parents have been separated, how well they know their new stepparent, whether they are being required to change schools or neighborhoods, and any other individual things that may be going on in their lives. They could even be contending with *two* new family situations if their other parent is in a relationship. It's a lot, and it can be complicated.

Parents can greatly up the odds for achieving blended family success if they:

☐ **Make time to connect.** Work to bond with your new, extended family members, and help stepsiblings to build relationships. This can mean starting new traditions – making hot cocoa on Saturday mornings, going on evening walks together, reading aloud from a favorite book. At the same time, be sure you and your spouse allow each other plenty of one-on-one time with your own children so nobody feels 'forgotten.' This crucial step can help alleviate the jealousy that can arise when there are new children competing for parents' time and attention.

☐ **Remain united.** Iron out a parenting strategy. Define what is expected of each parent in this new, blended scenario. In what situations or interactions should a stepparent get involved and when should they take a back seat? Do your best to follow consistent rules, homework plans and disciplinary policies. Be certain to include your ex-partner in this loop if the child spends time in their household. Kids are great at playing one against the other if given the opportunity. Try to be consistent across households and within your household.

☐ **Keep it to yourself.** Even under the most frustrating circumstances, try not to share negative remarks and feelings about your ex or your spouse's ex around your kids.

☐ **Know when to back off.** Earning the trust and respect of your new stepchildren takes time, sometimes years. Rushing in and expecting instant acceptance and love is unrealistic and attempting to take on a disciplinary role in order to earn respect is bound to backfire. Be the adult and give your relationship time to unfold and mature. If there is a lot of animosity, it may be time to bring in a therapist.

☐ **Embrace your place.** If you are a stepparent, view yourself as a "bonus." You aren't their parent, but you have a special position in their lives. You can be an advocate and trusted confidant.

☐ **Communicate constantly – with everyone.** Discuss and express emotions. Listen respectfully and encourage reciprocal communication.

You and your partner can also greatly improve your odds of forging a strong new family unit if you make these things priorities: treating each other with civility and respect, adapting to the different development levels of the kids involved, recognizing each other's experience levels as parents, and allowing space for growth and change.

Above all else, kids simply need to be reassured they are loved and secure within their new family dynamic.

## AMPLIFY YOUR EFFORTS.

Challenge yourself to maintain the most positive relationships possible with your child's other parent – in spite of past pain and conflict. Work to refocus. Your relationship with your ex should be a child-centered one, where the well-being of your kids – not your past hurts or resentment – is the primary focus. Past abuse or neglect on the part of an ex would certainly impact whether this is possible though. Safety always comes first!

Plan well ahead for family events like birthdays and holidays, and get the whole family involved. And be sure to coordinate with your ex to avoid last-second conflicts. Compromise is sure to be required. Work to keep things as equal as possible for all children – no big gifts or a party for one without reciprocal planning for all the others. Brainstorm to create new traditions for your blended family, something the kids can help plan and look forward to every year.

Finally, know when to seek help: If a child has unresolved anger toward a specific person, a step-parent openly favors one child over another, or it seems the family is struggling to function in a healthy way, turning to a therapist or other support person may be what is needed to get everyone back on track.

# RESOURCES:

Chertof J: *How to navigate challenges as a blended family*, December 2018. Available at: https://www.healthline.com/health/parenting/blended-family-tips

Huffington Post: *9 Strategies for making a blended family blend*. Available at:https://www.huffpost.com/entry/step-family-blended-family_n_6058890

Raising Children.net.au: *Blended families and children's feelings*. Available at: https://www.raisingchildren.net.au/grown-ups/family-diversity/blended-families-stepfamilies/feelings-about-blended-families

Robinson H: *A blended family united: Tips for overcoming issues together*. Available at: www.parents.com/parenting/divorce/blended-families/navigating-the-challenges-of-blended-families/ .

Segal J, Lawrence, L: *Blended family and step-parenting tips*. November, 2020. Available at: www.helpguide.org/articles/parenting-family/co-parenting-tips-for-divorced-parents.htm/.

# NOTES:

# 28

## KEEP FAMILY STORIES *Alive*

"I was born in Colombia, South America, while my husband comes from a large family of Americans with mixed European heritage. Together, we have two young children and are trying to provide them a sense of the richness of lives from both sides of the family. We want them to understand and value their roots."

We all come from somewhere – and we all come from somebody. A long line of somebodies, in fact. We've all got a back story that our kids should know and understand. Whether you hail from Cleveland, Caracas or Cairo, the stories, events and people that led to *you* are as complicated and circuitous as history itself.

Embracing your family history – recent and ancient, is part of creating family stability, but the ways family stories are shared look different for every family. Some families bond through cooking ethnic family recipes, speaking a shared language, or following certain religious or holiday traditions.

Telling stories about growing up on a dairy farm or surviving traumatic situations has the specific advantage of helping kids see how their family is unique and special. And there's evidence that kids who know their family history actually fare better in terms of solid coping skills, reduced anxiety and depression and feeling a stronger sense of connection.

Some key things to remember when sharing family history with your kids:

- Family stories are a big part of how we – and our relatives – will be remembered.
- Learning stories about extended family members can highlight them as heroes (it's not always about Mom or Dad!)
- Family stories help communicate family values.
- Listening to other people's stories honors them.

## PASS THE INFORMATION, PLEASE.

Building your kids' appreciation for where they came from is important to their sense of self – and self-esteem. Help make the process of learning about family fun through some of these family-focused activities:

☐ **Stories** – Ahh, the stories. Kids *love* them. So tell them about your high school antics (maybe with a few edits). Have grandma and grandpa tell them what life was like when they were kids, how they met and what their jobs were. What were new inventions when they were kids? Tell them about the struggles and the wins when you were a kid, the good stuff and the not-so-good stuff, how you faced problems and how you overcame them. It all adds up to a stronger sense of connection and belonging.

☐ **Scrapbooks** – Family photos are priceless. Looking at an album or scrapbook is like giving your kids and yourself a visual walk down memory lane. Being able to see the people and events that shaped your family give life to the stories you tell. Who knew your daughter looked just like her great aunt at four years old? So grandpa lived on a farm? Dad really played football? Give an empty scrapbook to the kids that they can fill with photos and items of interest to them.

☐ **Interviews** – Take the time to have your kids interview their relatives with a video recording. Let them pretend they are news reporters getting the action story for a TV show. Guide them in using the Who? What? When? Where? Why? format like actual reporters. Doing interviews at holidays or special family occasions can make these times even more meaningful for everyone around – even if they take place over Zoom. And interviewing different people about the same event can highlight how people remember and experience events in unique ways.

☐ **Map out a family tree or put together an online family history compendium.** Get help from the kids with the technical aspects as needed. Sort information by family member and family line – from Dad's side and Mom's side of the family. All kinds of data can be included – photos, documents, news items and more.

☐ **Make a memory matching game with pictures, events, stories.**

☐ **Find online news clippings of events related to the family.**

## AMPLIFY YOUR EFFORTS.

☐ If you are a parent of adopted children, be mindful of their heritage. If you know something about their ethnic or family history, make that part of your own family story and traditions. By showing an interest and commitment to learning their unique stories, you acknowledge that their background has value, is part of who they are, and is important to you too. Share what you can, always be willing to talk and support them through the issues that naturally come with this territory and remain open to helping them explore or investigate their family story when it is age and situation appropriate.

☐ Your family's roots are also based on culture. Talking with your kids about your family's traditions, foods, art and music, language, geographical origins, and histories of the places where family members came from enriches their sense of family. Take the time to share as much as you can about where your family came from.

## RESOURCES:

Reese E: What kids learn from hearing family stories. *The Atlantic*, December 9, 2013. Available at: http://www.theatlantic.com/education/archive/2013/12/what-kids-learn-from-hearing-family-stories/282075/.

Stuczynski A, Linik JR, Novick R: Family Stories, 2005. *Reading Rockets*. Available at: www.readingrockets.org/article/family-stories

## NOTES:

# PART THREE

## Safety

Safety: The extent to which a child is
free from fear of harm and secure from
physical or psychological harm within their
social and physical environment.[*]

Keeping kids safe is a team sport. It requires the adults in children's lives – parents, teachers, caregivers, coaches and other family members – to be invested in paying attention and intervening when needed to decrease the risk of harm. This book focuses heavily on the risks for physical and/or emotional abuse or neglect. But safety is a much broader topic that touches on everything from the food kids eat to their sleeping environment to the wider outside world filled with cars, bicycles, sports, activities, and school friends. It even extends to social media – where children can be emotionally harmed.

---

[*] Centers for Disease Control, National Center for Injury Prevention and Control, Division of Violence Prevention: *Essentials for Childhood: Creating Safe, Nurturing Relationships and Environments for All Children, 2019*

As kids grow and their lives expand into new environments, parents are called on to shift their thinking and approach in order to keep them safe. It's a tricky dance, but we've put together some tips to support you on the journey.

# 29
## Unplug

"Our family meals are always device-free affairs. Other times we disconnect are usually tied to vacation spots without cell coverage—in the mountains or at the beach—where there's no urge to check the phone and no disagreement about the urge to do so. I really look forward to our time to talk and not look at a screen, not answer the phone or respond to a text. Those things can wait. The time and conversation together are what's important."

I magine a doctor delivering the grim news that your child has a *"serious condition"* – one with a shockingly high chance of leading to behavioral disorders, anxiety, depression, sleep deprivation, emotional distress, poor nutrition and hygiene, disinterest in physical fitness, and challenges with relationships.

The cause of this disturbing diagnosis? Technology addiction. Your child, it appears, is incapable of prying his eyeballs away from the phone, TV or computer screen, and it's becoming a huge problem.

The numbers tell the story. The American Academy of Child and Adolescent Psychiatry (AACAP) reported in 2020 that on average, children 8-12 years old spent 4-6 hours a day watching or using screens, while teens spent up to nine hours. (And those numbers didn't count online learning hours related to COVID.)

Make no mistake, technology addiction is leading children and adults down a slippery slope that is contributing to soaring rates of physical and emotional distress. It's interfering with their ability to be productive and enjoy the present, where they can be surrounded by real people in real situations in real time.

The benefits of taking a break from technology can be remarkable. One study conducted by UCLA revealed that sixth graders who went just 5 days without their devices were much better able to read human emotions than those who did not.

It's hard to imagine our world without technology. Increasingly simple and powerful electronic devices offer instant access to friends, facts, news and entertainment—which is immensely appealing. It's not all bad, either. Social and educational content available on television, computers, cell phones, and even wrist watches can be especially helpful to children with emotional, intellectual, and physical challenges.

But for all its benefits, technology has some major drawbacks – beyond the time it steals. Exposure to violence and other inappropriate content can be dangerous. The consequences are especially harmful for younger children whose growing bodies and brains just aren't equipped to handle it. The AACAP notes that children may be exposed to violence and risk-taking behaviors, sexual content, negative stereotypes, substance abuse, cyberbullies and predators (25% of teenagers say they've been bullied either by text or on the internet), and misleading or inaccurate information.

For older kids, many risky behaviors are rooted in the misuse of technology—particularly internet pornography. In 82% of online sex crimes against children, sex offenders used social networking sites to gain information about their victims. Children themselves often unwittingly share inappropriate content with their peers. Nearly a quarter of 14 -17-year-olds report having participated in some sort of nude sexting (JAMA Pediatrics, 2020). Many teens may be unaware that sharing nude photos of children is considered a crime. Make sure they are informed!

## FINDING THE BALANCE.

Back to our original diagnosis. "So, doctor," you would immediately ask upon being delivered this news. "Is there something – *anything* – I can do to help my child?"

And this is where things get dicey. Because yes, there is a cure. But it can be painful for kids to endure and difficult for parents to enforce. That's because the only known remedy for this condition is to take intermittent breaks from technology. Tone down the texting, unwire the wi-fi, put an end to unlimited computer time, and ditch the Xbox. In other words, unplug.

Implementing the eight suggestions below can help to strike a balance between complete device absorption and interacting with the world. The kids are going to gripe at first, guaranteed. Let them.

The stakes are too high to back down.

☐ **Limit the use of TV, computers and mobile devices.** Here are some AACAP guidelines on what is considered reasonable, broken down by age:

Less than 18 months: Only video chatting with an adult present

18-24 months: Educational programming watched with a caregiver

2-5 years: Limit non-educational time to one hour per weekday and three hours on weekend days

6 years and older: Encourage healthy habits and limit activities that include screens.

☐ **Schedule an appropriate time for using devices, and plan fun physical activities for your child to engage in at other times.** Get outside! Ride a bike! Build a fort! Take a walk!

☐ **Refrain from putting TV and electronic gadgets in your** child's bedroom, and put away such devices after use. Turn off screens 30-60 minutes before bedtime.

☐ **Observe 'tech-free' times during meals, homework, and bedtime**. In addition, designate 'tech-free' zones in your home. Have kids check their phones in and out with you when doing homework or at bedtime.

☐ **Teach your child early about the importance of moderation**. Be sure to offer praise when your child demonstrates restraint in the use of tech devices and follows the rules you've set.

☐ **Monitor access by using the device together with your child.** Take this opportunity to communicate, interact, and share family values. With teens, this suggestion is more difficult but communication is more critical than ever in these years. Continue to share your values and make it your business to know about the kinds of websites they visit and social media they use. Above all, make it clear that you're paying attention.

☐ **Talk, talk, talk to maximize the advantages and minimize the disadvantages of technology.** This goal requires both education and monitoring. Talk with your kids about what's appropriate with regard to both content and daily use, no matter their age. Be sure teens know about the danger of interacting with strangers online and the ways in which kids can be recruited into sex trafficking.

Taking breaks from technology is not only a healthy goal—it's a *necessity* for children. The cost is small, and the potential rewards are priceless. Better sleep, better grades, more reading, more active time, fewer mood problems, and more time learning alternative ways to relax and have fun are all benefits.

## AMPLIFY YOUR EFFORTS.

You're all set to lay down the limits with your kids, which is fantastic. Now it's time to take a look at your own habits.

Be honest with yourself and your susceptibility to what some call "digital heroin." How many hours do *you* spend online, texting, checking e-mail or scrolling through Facebook, Instagram, TikTok, Twitter? How many times have you had a near-miss with a power pole while you simultaneously walked and texted? And how much of that do your kids witness?

Try resisting temptation the next time you feel the urge. Pocket your own phone, shut your laptop, and be present. Your kids will benefit!

---

# RESOURCES:

American Academy of Child and Adolescent Psychiatry: *Screen time and children*. Number 51, February 2020.

Becker J: *9 Important strategies for raising children in a world of technology*, 2017. Available at: www.becomingminimalist.com/ikids/.

Ehmke R: *Media guidelines for kids of all ages*, n.d. Child Mind Institute. Available at: http://www.childmind.org/article/media-guidelines-for-kids-of-all-ages/
(Also in Spanish)

Hurley K: *Teen sexting: what parents need to know.* 2021. Available at: http://www.psycom.net/teen-sexting/

Jeglic E: *Teen sexting: Guidelines for parents*, 2020. Available at: http://www.psychologytoday.com/us/blog/protecting-children-sexual-abuse/202001/teen-sexting-guidelines-parents.

# NOTES:

# 30

# *Call* IT LIKE IT IS –
# BODY PARTS HAVE NAMES

"In 20 years of pediatric practice—both in primary care and child abuse—I continue to be amazed by the degree to which children and teens struggle to identify and talk about their private areas. I used to spend a great deal of time during well-child visits trying to normalize the terms vagina, penis, buttocks, and breasts, encouraging parents to use them when talking with their children at home. It's extremely difficult to understand a child's specific issue (or address concerns of sexual abuse) when they identify both vagina and buttocks as "privates" or worse, use slang such as "kooka" or "winky." Giving children the correct names and permission to talk about their private areas helps them communicate their serious concerns to us."

Raise your hand if you know what a "tootie" is. No? How about a coochie? A piddlewiddle?

If not, don't feel bad. Spell-checker doesn't recognize them either. For the record, all three are slang for body parts usually covered by pants.

Why is it that we call a child's foot a foot, her ear an ear, his mouth a mouth—yet continue to avoid using appropriate terms for their

147

penises and vaginas? The answer may go a long way toward helping immunize children to sexual abuse that's rooted in a lack of awareness and secrecy surrounding their genitals.

Pediatricians and child development experts say using slang references for body parts can undermine children's physical, social, and sexual development. They also play into the hands of sexual predators, who know how to take advantage of their victim's lack of awareness and whose abuse is shrouded in discomfort and secrecy.

So parents, be aware. It's critical to teach your children about *every* part of their body—in ways that are developmentally and culturally appropriate. It takes practice. And it may never be perfect. But it will definitely help – and help *protect* – our kids for years to come.

## BE CLEAR.

Take a deep breath and shake off your own embarrassment. Then tackle this first order of business: ***Teach young kids that their "private parts" (covered by a bathing suit) are off limits to other people.*** Emphasizing this helps to minimize shame and maximize both their awareness and sense of control.

This knowledge also helps kids become more comfortable around medical issues and examinations, resist unwanted or inappropriate overtures, and talk more freely and accurately in the unfortunate event of a violation.

One of the most effective tools for preventing abuse is taking the stigma off the names. Feeling a little awkward? We're here to help:

**Let pictures do the talking**. Picture books go a long way toward breaking down the awkwardness of this topic, and can be especially effective with younger children. *(See Resources for suggestions).* Point out body parts and name them.

**Remember that consistency and accuracy are crucial**. Some families may speak a language other than English, and the names for body parts may reflect their primary language. For others, "vagina" or "penis" may be uncomfortable words. That's OK. Perhaps "boy's front private" and "girl's front private" feels more natural. The key is to use words that accurately describe the body part in question.

Know that teaching children the correct names for their reproductive body parts helps them to develop a healthier, more positive body image while better equipping them to understand their bodies and ask questions about sexual development.

## AMPLIFY YOUR EFFORTS.

- Ask other family members or caregivers who spend time with your kids to be consistent with the vocabulary you choose to use.

Be part of the movement working to protect children by sharing your knowledge on the topic with others. Reinforce the message that the anatomically correct terminology for any body part is never a "bad word." As the American Academy of Pediatrics explains, it's vital to teach that genitals, while private, "are not so private that you can't talk about them."

---

# RESOURCES:

Buni C: *The case for teaching kids 'vagina,' 'penis,' and 'vulva,'* 2013. Available at: www.theatlantic.com/health/archive/2013/04/the-case-for-teaching-kids-vagina-penis-and-vulva/274969/.

Matthews D: *Call children's private body parts what they are*, 2017. Available at: www.psychologytoday.com/blog/going-beyond-intelligence/201703/call-children-s-private-body-parts-what-they-are.

Starishevsky J: *My body belongs to me.* Available at: www.mybodybelongstome.com/.

# NOTES:

# 31

## Don't Panic
### IF THEY "PLAY DOCTOR"

"I can remember 'playing doctor' with my best friend, Janie, when we were about five years old. We took turns in the doctor role, carefully examining each other's bodies, including our private parts. Janie had three younger sisters, so perhaps it wasn't so enlightening for her, but I had two younger brothers so looking at little girl parts was very new to me. Janie's mother interrupted our role playing in an easy way. I don't think she was worried that we were doing anything unsafe, but many parents worry that perhaps this exploration is the beginning of problematic sexual behavior or just not the right thing for little kids to do. I don't remember this sexual exploration occurring more than that one time."

Curiosity is a huge part of what makes us human. Truly, if we didn't ask questions *all the time* where we would be as a species? Certainly not sitting in comfortable homes with central heating, scrolling on our smart phones. When you're fairly new to the world, everything comes with huge question marks: *What does this do? How does that work? What if…? I wonder what…?* Even before our brains have the language to form questions, we are driven to learn.

Natural curiosity is all about gathering information and learning – and kids have a lot to learn when it comes to sexuality. It starts at a basic level. What are our body parts? What are they called? What are they for? What are the differences between boys and girls? How are babies made? Kids want to *know*. And they learn a ton by watching, asking questions, receiving feedback from others, and trying countless new things. Learning about sexual functions is a normal developmental step.

Among those countless things kids will question and try in their lifetimes, early sexual exploration – or "playing doctor" – is extremely common. So if you happen to stumble upon your child doing just that, take a deep breath. It's okay.

Still, it's only natural for a child's sexual development and exploration to spark questions in adults about what, exactly, is developmentally appropriate and what is an indicator of a child who is at risk for sexual problems? Why do some kids seem more "advanced" and others less so?

The answer is complicated. All kinds of factors come into the picture when evaluating the nature of a young child's sexual exploration. The environment that a child is raised in, religious and cultural norms, family living spaces and opportunities for privacy, number and age of siblings, level of daily supervision, the media, and other children all play the media, other children – they all play a part in the sexual development of kids.

Children whose parents argue about sex, tell sexual jokes, make sexual gestures, watch pornography when kids are around, or make sexual comments about others' bodies are at higher risk for developing problematic sexual behaviors. And there are plenty of other risk factors, including family stress, poverty, rejection and family violence.

## SO, IS IT INNOCENT...OR NOT?

When it comes to sexual behaviors and curiosity in school-age children, what's nothing to worry about and when should you be more concerned?

**For children in kindergarten through fourth grade, healthy sexual curiosity might be that they:**

- Ask questions about sexual body parts, their functions, gender differences, and making babies.
- Are interested in bathroom functions and sexual behavior.
- Touch their own genitals when settling for sleep, excited or stressed, or just because it "feels good."
- Use "dirty" language for bathroom and sexual functions and make jokes using such words.
- Play games using parent roles – such as pretending to have a baby. If the child is at the younger end of the age group or if the role playing is quite specific for adult behavior, this may be cause for concern. Seek advice.
- Want privacy.
- Look at and touch the genitals, breasts, or buttocks of others if they are preschoolers.
- Kiss and hug familiar children and adults and allow reciprocal behavior.
- May look at pictures of people in the nude or draw genitalia for human figures.

**Causes for concern:**

- Repeatedly or consistently exhibit behaviors, language, or concerns regarding bodies, their functions, and sexual roles.
- Use "dirty" words even after consistently being told "no" and may have been disciplined for using these words.
- Repeatedly play "doctor" or mimic sexual behavior with other children or dolls. Force sexual contact or games on another child or adult.
- Show or rub genitals in public after being told "no" repeatedly. Show genitals at school or in other places to express anger.
- Use sex talk that gets them in trouble. Romanticize or sexualize relationships.
- Want to play sexual games with much older, younger

(three-year difference is rule-of-thumb), or unfamiliar children.
- Want to see genitals or breasts of others, sneak peeks or make others feel uncomfortable.
- Exhibit sexual behaviors with animals.
- Draw human figures with exaggerated genitalia or compulsively look at videos or other media of nudity that get the child into trouble.

Other concerning behaviors include:

- Threatening other children not to tell
- Invasive or penetrating sexual contact

## SO WHAT'S A PARENT TO DO?

For children of all ages, the American Academy of Pediatrics has these recommendations for parents:

☐ **Use appropriate language for the names of body parts**. Kids need to know the same names for body parts that other people use in order to communicate with them. Also teach what parts are "private" (covered by a swimming suit).

☐ **Make sure to respect the modesty of both adults and children and teach your children to be respectful too**. At around five years old, children start to develop their own sense of modesty.

☐ **Explain safe versus unsafe touch**. Safe touch is a way for people to say they care for each other and help each other. Unsafe touch is touch that is not wanted. Kids need to learn they should say "no" to unsafe touch and tell you about situations that are confusing or scary to them. **It is *never* okay for anyone to look at or touch their private parts**. The only exception is the doctor or nurse who has a parent nearby when they need to help the child get well or stay healthy.

☐ **Control media exposure.** Use parental controls available through internet providers. Know the rating systems for video games, movies, and television shows and use that information to choose appropriate media for kids to watch. Supervise viewing time and what is being watched. Talk with your child about what they are watching and playing. Stay connected with their internet and device use.

☐ **Answer questions honestly and respectfully, even if the question seems cute or weird or unexpected.** Be brief with answers. Let the child ask the next question if he or she wants to know more. Say, "Does that answer your question?" Respond based on your child's reaction.

☐ **Gently guide your child's sexual curiosity and behaviors**: For example, "We only do that in private." Or, "It looks like you're interested in seeing each other's private parts. Let's look at a book that has pictures of private parts together." "These are my private parts. Please don't touch them, and remember that no one should touch your private parts." And be sure to tell them: "If anyone does this to you, tell a parent or trusted adult" so that they don't feel guilty for "letting it happen" if they are abused.

☐ **Always try to react calmly, redirect when necessary or increase supervision if you find your kids engaging in sexual behaviors –** whether developmentally appropriate or concerning. Your responses to your child's questions and actions can help them to develop normal, healthy sexual attitudes, values, and behaviors.

## AMPLIFY YOUR EFFORTS.

☐ **If your child exhibits concerning sexual behaviors, don't be shy about talking with your pediatric primary care provider.** You can also call a mental health specialist familiar with child sexuality issues. For a referral, reach out to a community mental health center, university counseling center, pediatrician, hospital or the Child Advocacy Center in your area (which can provide support regarding cases of abuse and neglect of children in your specific community).

☐ **If you suspect that your child is in danger due to sexual abuse, call child protective services and/or the police.** You might also reach out to the National Child Abuse Hotline, (1-800-4-A-CHILD) or you may have a hotline exclusive to your state.

Anytime you have concerns, ask for help!

## RESOURCES:

American Academy of Pediatrics: *Sexual behaviors in young children: What's normal, what's not?* Available at: https://www. Healthychildren.org/English/ages-stages/preschool/Pages/Sexual-Behaviors-Young-Children.aspx.

De Bruin, K: *Childhood Sexual Exploration vs. Childhood Sexual Abuse*, June 8, 2018. Available at: https://www.kathryndebruin. com/2018/06/08/signs-of-abuse/

Johnson, TC: *Understanding Children's Sexual Behaviors: What's Natural and Healthy.* www.tcavjohn.com, 2015. (Website)

Johnson, TC. *Updated-Helping children with sexual behavior problems: A guidebook for professionals and caregivers,* 4th ed. www.tcavjohn.com, 2016. See website above.

National Children's Alliance: *Effective Treatment for Youth with Problematic Sexual Behaviors.* (See National Children's Alliance website).

# NOTES:

# 32

# *Know* YOUR KIDS' COACHES, TEACHERS AND MENTORS

"I was very active in track and field in high school and college and worked with lots of coaches along the way. Most were wonderful, supportive, encouraging people who helped me achieve my goals, but there was one who took advantage of his role as a powerful person in my life and was abusive. It was so hard for me as a young person. I felt that I didn't have a choice since he was in charge of my athletic development and achievement. I kept the secret of my abuse for much of my life but eventually recognized that I needed professional help and spent many years in therapy, healing. I'm committed to teaching coaches and parents how to avoid these kinds of situations."

The second we drop our kids off at school, sports or music practice, we're entrusting their safety and well-being to other adults. As a parent, that takes guts – and no small measure of trust.

Many kids spend countless hours in the company of coaches, teachers, scout leaders and others who are in positions of power. These mentors can be among the most impactful people in a child's life. Good mentors for kids understand that responsibility, want the best for their students, and work hard to establish boundaries that are safe for everyone. But you've seen the headlines. Just as in any other area of life, not all mentors for kids are good people.

Studies show that 2-8% of athletes become victims of abuse by a coach or teacher, which is clearly 2-8% too many. Violators may be young, old, married, single, parents or childless. Most are male, but some offenders are women. An abuser's strategy is usually to seek out a vulnerable child, build trust and eventually exploit their authority by crossing the boundary into a sexual relationship with the young person. They work to be sure the young person will cooperate and keep the relationship secret, reflecting the power they have. The same thing can happen to kids at camps, in scouts, or other activities.

Although sexual abuse receives the most attention, abuse can be physical, emotional, or involve bullying, either by adults or other kids involved with the activity. Being aware and alert to the adults in your child's orbit is critical.

## COVER YOUR BASES.

It's impossible to have eyes on your child 24/7, but there are steps you can take to protect your family and learn as much as possible about the people you entrust them to.

☐ **Conduct background checks.** Ensure your sports league or activity group has a policy to conduct annual background checks on all coaches and volunteers.

☐ **Establish a code of conduct.** Whether it's a team or family policy, put safeguards in place; for example, screening – or not allowing – individual texts between people in authority and youth.

☐ **Enforce strength in numbers.** Make sure there are multiple adults supervising children, and never allow one-on-one interactions. If you can be at practices, meetings or events, show up and make your presence known.

☐ **Keep it out in the open.** Insist that there be no interactions between adults and children behind closed doors. Everything should be observable by parents or other adults.

☐ **No socializing.** Individualized attention outside of regularly scheduled activities where others are present should never happen.

☐ **Get trained.** Demand that adults who work with kids in your area or school district be regularly trained on issues related to child abuse and neglect. One program to explore: Darkness to Light's "Stewards of Children" sexual abuse prevention training. (See Resources below.)

☐ **At home, teach your kids about acceptable and unacceptable behavior or attention from adults – or anyone, for that matter.** Let them know that they should tell you any time they feel uncomfortable around an adult and that "keeping secrets" with another adult is never okay.

☐ **Be attentive to changes in your child's behavior that could indicate trauma:** nightmares, depression, desire to avoid activities they used to like, or reduced self-esteem.

☐ **If you suspect an adult who works with kids is being abusive, take action.** But never blame the child! (See Tip #36 – Don't Blame the Victim.) Report the situation to your pediatric health care provider, the police, the District Attorney's office, or your Child Abuse Advocacy Center (National Hotline number: 1-800-422-4453).

## AMPLIFY YOUR EFFORTS.

Parents are often recruited to coach teams or lead Scouts or other activities for their young kids – which is generous, inspiring, and life-changing for many children.

Should you choose to mentor kids, protect yourself. Follow

the tips above: never be alone with a young person, communicate directly with parents or with the group, recruit an assistant to ensure an extra layer of safety and get trained on safe practices.

Coaches, teachers, scout leaders, and other mentors can change the world. Make sure those changes are all positive.

# RESOURCES:

Darkness to Light: *5 Steps to Protecting Children* 2017. Available at: https://www.d2l.org/education/5-steps/ (Website). (Available in many languages).

De Lench B: *Abuse in youth sports takes many different forms*. 2018. Mom's Team. Available at: https://www.momsteam.com/health-safety/emotional-injuries/general/abuse-in-youth-sports-takes-many-different-forms

Parent S, El Hlimi K: *Sexual Abuse of Young People in Sport, Institut national de sante publique Quebec*, 2012. Available at: www.inspq.qc.ca/en/sexual-assault/fact-sheets/sexual-abuse-young-people-sport (Also in French).

Small FL: *Combating Sexual Abuse in Youth Sports*, January 6, 2018. Available at: www.psychologytoday.com/us/blog/coaching-and-parenting-young-athletes/201801/combating-sexual-abuse-in-youth-sports.

Thomas S & LaBotz M: *Preventing abuse in youth sports and organized activities*. 2018. AAP, Healthy Children. Available at: https://www.healthychildren.org/English/healthy-living/sports/Pages/Preventing-Abuse-in-Youth-Sports-and-Organized-Activities.aspx (Also in Spanish)

# NOTES:

# 33

## *Banish* BULLIES

"When I taught second graders, I had one student who was light years ahead of her classmates academically and socially. But as the year progressed, her work began to slip and she became withdrawn. I checked in with her parents regularly—but nobody could seem to figure out what was going on. One day, she began sobbing and disclosed that she had been teased by a couple of classmates ever since she had gotten glasses. Everything immediately got better once she was consoled and given some advice about how to address the culprits. It's important to remember that children internalize things differently and may not know how to process the experience of being bullied, regardless of severity. Adults should prioritize teaching children about the issue at an early age to mitigate the impact of any bullying or teasing that they experience or witness."

- You're five years old, and you don't mind saying you've got your kindergarten routine down cold. But when a new student transfers into your classroom, the other kids don't waste a second before starting to pick on him. You know it doesn't feel right, but what can you do?

- You're in middle school – unofficial lifetime headquarters of social awkwardness. School can be stressful, due, in no small measure, to to the kid who sits next to you in English class, and has decided YOU are the next player on *"Who can I harass now? And while I'm at it, let's do it every single day!"* You're afraid to speak up for fear it will just make everything worse.

- You're a high school sophomore aching for popularity, and you're pretty sure calling a few people out on social media is just the ticket to get some much-needed laughs and attention.

- Now let's say you're a parent, and your child has been one – or maybe all – of these kids: an observer, a victim, or a perpetrator of bullying. What are YOU going to do?

Let's be clear on what bullying is: *unwanted, aggressive behavior that involves a real or perceived power imbalance.*

"Bullying" has been a buzzword for a number of years now, which may account for recent studies which suggest the problem is improving. Yet, about one in five children still experience some form of bullying, Thirty percent of kids admit to having bullied other children, and over 70% have witnessed others being bullied. For many children, being a witness to or victim of this behavior can be difficult to process.

Bullying victims are at risk for physical injuries, psychological distress, and even suicide. Identity-based bullying, particularly toward LGBTQ+ youth, is prevalent and more strongly correlated with negative outcomes than bullying in general.

## SO, WHAT ARE YOU GOING TO DO ABOUT IT?

Plenty, we hope. Clearly, it's impossible to watch our kids around the clock and schools generally frown upon full-time parental escorts or bodyguards. But we can – and should – continue to teach our kids how to treat others right and how to protect themselves. The old adage of "turn the other cheek" doesn't cut it. Kids need to be equipped to address bullying head-on in order to minimize negative impacts.

Some techniques for kids who are being bullied:

- [ ] **Ask the bully to STOP—loudly if necessary.**

- [ ] **Look the bully in the eyes and laugh – even hysterical laughter, which works by disarming the bully.** Another approach? Look the person in the eyes and respond by being nice.

- [ ] **Walk away – nonchalance, as if the bully was a stranger.**

- [ ] **Talk to a trusted adult to share what is happening and form a plan for handling it.**

- [ ] **Make an effort to be around others.** Typically, bullying occurs when adults are not around.

- [ ] **Recognize that bullies are attempting to steal power.** If the victim acts unintimidated, the bully may lose interest.

What KIDS can do to help prevent bullying:

- [ ] **Treat others with respect.** Remember that we are all different – not "better" or "worse."

- [ ] **Stand up for others.** Report incidents of bullying to a trusted adult like a teacher or parent.

- [ ] **Treat kids who are being bullied with kindness.** Sit by them and include them in other activities.

- [ ] **Protect themselves from cyberbullying.** This means 'think before posting,' don't share passwords, and be on the alert about what is seen online.

What YOU can do:

- [ ] **Encourage children to speak to a trusted adult if they witness or experience bullying.** Seek help if your child is experiencing significant bullying, which is categorized as abuse.

☐ Talk with school officials or call the Child Abuse Hotline if any child is at risk.

☐ Talk with a mental health provider if a child is not coping with bullying by others.

☐ Check in with your kids often to gain a better understanding of their concerns.

☐ Model how to treat others with kindness and respect.

☐ Monitor your kids' social media accounts and educate yourself about cyberbullying.

☐ Visit stopbullying.gov for more information on how to address and prevent bullying. (See Chapter 35 for more on this topic).

☐ Be supportive rather than controlling to keep your kid from engaging in cyberbullying. Being supportive means considering the child's perspective while working to guide the child to do the right thing.

## AMPLIFY YOUR EFFORTS:

Want to make a real difference in your area or school? Encourage your kids to make sure teachers, counselors and others know what is going on in school by sharing information about what they see and hear.

If your children are truly motivated, help them speak up and start or join an anti-bullying campaign. Plan an assembly or invite a guest speaker to school who can speak to everyone about bullying.

# RESOURCES:

Earnshaw VA, Juvonen J, Reisner SL, et al: LGBTQ bullying: translating research to action in pediatrics. *Pediatrics* 140(4): e20170432, 2017

McCleary E: *Parenting strategies linked to teen cyberbullying behavior,* 2021. Teens and Tech. Available at: http://www.teensandtech.org/the-latest-science/parenting-strategies-linked-to-teen-cyberbullying-behavior

NYU News: Teens who think their parents are loving are less likely to cyberbully. Available at: https://www.nyu.edu/about/news-publications/news/2020/september/teens-cyberbullying.html

Strasburger V, Zimmerman H, Temple JR, et al: *Teens, Sexting, and the Law,* 2019. Pediatrics 45(143)5, May 2019, e220183183

Stomp Out Bullying: *How to deal with bullies: what to do.* Available at: www.stompoutbullying.org/get-help/about-bullying-and-cyberbullying/are-you-being-bullied.

U.S. Department of Health and Human Services (USDHHS): *Get help now.* Available at: www.stopbullying.gov website. (Also in Spanish).

Waasdorp TE, Pas ET, Zablotsky B, et al: Ten-year trends in bullying and related attitudes among 4th- to 12th- graders, *Pediatrics* 139(6): e20162615, 2017.

# NOTES:

# 34
## *Be* THE CHANGE

"Our family is Black and we live in a city that is not very racially diverse. With two kids in middle school, it hurts me to think about them being exposed to racial slurs or other treatment that could affect their self-esteem. I want them to feel proud of who they are in every way! So we work hard to educate them about our family history and cultural roots, as well as teach them tools for educating others and managing any negative messages that may be directed toward them."

Prejudice. Bias. Racism. They're triple threats to the safety and health of our communities. We've all witnessed racist behavior in action; the most egregious examples grab headlines on a daily basis, sometimes involving people who are considered powerful or privileged.

Let's break it down:

- *Prejudice* is a preconceived opinion that is not based on reason or actual experience. Pre-judged.

- *Bias* is prejudice in favor of or against one thing, person, or group compared with another, usually in a way considered to be unfair. Let's be clear. We *all* carry biases within us. It's just part of our human condition, but one we can work to improve.

- *Racism* is the belief that groups of humans possess different behavioral traits corresponding to inherited attributes and can be divided based on the superiority of one group over another.

If there is a hierarchy, racism would be like the chest-thumping school bully, with prejudice and bias its loyal sidekicks, knocking people down a notch with casual comments, blanket assumptions, social exclusions. You know – a jab here, a snub there. We call these micro-aggressions. And although they may seem small, their overall impact is tremendous.

Racism always has – and continues to – split our society in some pretty terrible ways. Racial slurs, words and actions marginalize others, damage self-esteem, and can affect the ability of all people to lead just as good a life as anyone else. Bias, prejudices, and racist beliefs say to another person: "You are 'other' in a way I don't respect, and your otherness automatically makes you lesser than me." That otherness encompasses skin color, cultural background, language, or religion. The list could go on: gender, sexual orientation, financial status, education level and so much more.

Maybe you or your family have never been a target. Perhaps you have never feared sending your child out into the world, knowing they are more likely to encounter violence or hateful comments based purely on the color of their skin. Or be ridiculed for getting free lunch at school. Or excluded because of a perceived (or actual) disability. But maybe you or your family has experienced it personally.

Racism hurts all of us. So how can we equip our kids to:

a) learn not to think, believe, or behave in exclusionary ways;
b) develop, grow, and thrive despite the racism that flares around them;
c) become adults who will recognize and embrace differences, and do what they can to eliminate the perpetuation of racist values and ideals?

Our work as parents starts early. By age two, kids will begin to notice differences among people – skin and hair, eye shape and color, disabilities. More verbal three and four-year-olds may ask questions like "Why is your skin that color?" Five-year-olds will begin to identify ethnic groups and can point out more detailed similarities and differences among people.

Children learn racism and prejudice from the adults around them from an early age. But hate and intolerance can also be unlearned. Raising confident and caring children means equipping them with the knowledge that they deserve love and respect. Tackling racism involves instilling children with the desire to understand other people and the grit to go out in the world and stand up for those who are different.

This is hard stuff, and no, none of it is fair. But we're human, and we simply don't know what it's like to be something or someone other than who we are. Often, we operate on fear or suspicion of what we don't know. But we can try harder. We can train ourselves, and our kids, to not automatically 'assume.' We can keep an open mind and we can learn. If we want to build a more loving and positive world for our kids, there's important work to be done.

## RISE ABOVE.

Talk, talk and talk some more. Kids aren't color blind, and they don't have to be. Differences are not only okay, but 100 percent real and unavoidable. Talk about them positively! And get ready for the questions. *Why is her hair blue? Why is your skin a different color? Is that person a man or a woman? Why is my hair curly and yours is straight?* And so on.

Some other ways you can prepare your kids to fight prejudice and pursue acceptance:

☐ **Work to create experiences rich with variety,** including music, language, and food from places around the world. Choose a different country or ethnicity to explore each month, preparing food, watching movies, reading books, and listening to music that is representative of that culture. And challenge yourself to not reinforce stereotypes, instead exploring the variety of customs, people, and activities that exist within every culture.

☐ **Draw on the strengths of your family background.** Tell stories of resistance, resilience, and joy. Do you have grand-parents or other family members who can share history? This is the kind of stuff that binds a family together and creates a sense of pride and belonging. Tap into that power.

☐ **Read books and watch movies or shows with characters from diverse backgrounds.** Here's an opportunity to show you value diversity. Discuss the characters and welcome your kids' questions. Teens can certainly delve into richer reading material that can crack open entirely new worlds. If they're open to it, help guide them by researching and recommending appropriate choices.

☐ **Discuss differences within groups of people.** For example, the word "Asian" represents people from almost 50 different countries – all with their own customs, languages, religions, foods and beliefs. Being mindful not to lump everyone into a broad category is an important step in recognizing people's individuality.

☐ **Dive into our own culture as Americans.** What are some of the things we do that are particular to our culture but may be different from others? What things do we do that exclude others and what do we do that is inclusive?

☐ **Work to push outside your comfort zone.** Pursue diversity in where you choose to live, the schools you select for your kids, and the toys they play with. Diversify and expand your circle of friends, and help your kids do the same.

☐ **Be prepared to act.** Silence signals acceptance to children. If you hear or witness something inappropriate, be prepared to speak up. Within your own home, set a zero-tolerance policy for name calling, mocking, or disrespecting others. Get help if your child is experiencing trauma from racism.

## AMPLIFY YOUR EFFORTS.

Racism (and prejudice) is a heavy topic, and an ongoing story. You can dive further into these issues by:

- ☐ **Being a historian.** Read, ask questions, and expand your own knowledge of bigotry and oppression among various religions and ethnicities throughout history. What are some of the racial problems we have faced in this country and how are we trying to address them?

- ☐ **Talking about legal injustice with your children.** Just because some laws or local rules might not exist doesn't mean racial or biased acts are right. Teach them that when brave people speak up about problems and ask for better treatment of all people, things can change for the better.

- ☐ **Nurturing your kids to become critical thinkers.** Delve deeper into stories of race in books, movies, and in the media. Discuss things like: Who is speaking? Why? How does that fit with what you know? Who was hurt by another person's words or actions? What could have been done differently?

Remember that this is a topic where the conversation will never end. Keep after it.

---

## RESOURCES:

Abdullah M: How adults can support the mental health of Black children. Available at: https://greatergood.berkeley.edu/article/item/how_adults_can_support_mental_health_black_children

EmbraceRace: *16 ways to help children become thoughtful, informed, and brave about race* 2021. Available at: https://www.embracerace.org/resources/16-ways-to-help-children-become-thoughtful-informed-and-brave-about-race (Also in Spanish)

Jewish Federation of Greater New Haven: *Resources for discussions about racism, inclusion and justice.* Available at: https://jewishnewhaven.org/George-floyd/resources

Mack LE: *9 Resources for non-black parents of Black children, recommended by experts.* Available at: https://www.romper.com/p/9-resources-for-non-black-parents-of-black-children-recommended-by-experts-families-22979648

Mostafa B: *Raising race-conscious children: How to talk to kids about race and racism,* 2020. From University of Michigan Health. Available at: https://healthblog.uofmhealth.org/childrens-health/raising-race-conscious-children-how-to-talk-to-kids-about-race-and-racism

Oleson N: *How to talk to your white kids about racism.* Jewish Family Services. Available at:https://www.jfcsmpls.org/how-to-talk-to-your-white-kids-about-racism

Rodriguez C: Talking with young children about bias and prejudice. Anti-Defamation League. Available at: www.adl.org/education/resources/tools-and-strategies/talking-to-young-children-about-prejudice

---

# NOTES:

# 35

## KEEP THE "SOCIAL" IN
# Social Media

> "We live in an age where we eat, breathe, and live the internet and social media. Having the world at our fingertips is intoxicating and powerful, yet we entrust it to the hands of younger and younger children. We're good at teaching kids how to be polite and pleasant in the real world, but somehow forget to teach them how to act when they focus on the screens they are glued to."

It's 9 p.m. Do you know where your kids are? Odds are they're just down the hall, studying... or something. And *of course*, they've got their cell phone/iPad /laptop glued to them because, well, attempting to function without those is akin to removing a vital body part. All of which is to say that, sure, the kids may be physically down the hall. But they also have the entire universe at their fingertips, and that's a very scary notion, indeed.

There was a time not long ago, when pre-teens and teens had the freedom to make unwise decisions and impulsive moves without those actions being preserved forevermore on a camera, video, or text message. Social media has thrown all of that out the window. Now, all it takes is half a second and a "send" button to

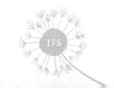

impact somebody's world, whether that means being self-destructive or destructive of others.

The Internet and social media can be powerful – and enriching – when used appropriately. But even teens know those tools are risky, with many reporting they spend too much time on their cell phone and on social media. Widely cited research from the Pew Center showed that 45% of teens reported they were online "almost constantly." The most frequently reported reason for feeling negative about social media was the likelihood of bullying or rumor spreading.

Teaching children early about how and when to take advantage of these tools, while being mindful of how their words and actions impact others, is critical. It's never too early. As soon as your child starts talking, you can begin laying the groundwork for positive online – and offline – habits.

## BE THE BOSS OF "YOUR" INTERNET.

We don't call it "the Web" for nothing. The Internet – and social media – is a place where even the most grounded among us can get lost. You might be sitting across the breakfast table from your child and have absolutely zero idea what messages they are reading, seeing, sending or absorbing

That's the age we live in. We can't roll back the clock to 1990, so as parents, what *can* we do?

☐ **Know the playing field.** Make it your business to know what social media tools and apps are out there. Kids are *waaaayyyy* ahead of most adults on this curve. In fact, if parents or adults are using a particular type of social media, kids and teens have probably already moved on to a new one.

☐ **Join them.** Open your own account on the sites your kids are on so you'll have a better idea of what's up.

☐ **Become an expert before your child does.** Before you hand your kid a cell phone, research. Learn about popular tools or sites that attract kids. How do they operate? What parental controls do they offer or lack and what are their age requirements? Remember, children learn quickly and if you aren't there to teach them, they will get their information elsewhere. This is your opportunity to lay solid groundwork about family expectations and how to behave online.

☐ **Don't assume anything.** Your kids are likely to have more than one social media account, sometimes under different names, and may not understand how vulnerable they are or how to protect themselves. Consistently drive home the importance of never giving out personal information (full name, address, school name, age, etc.) to anyone they don't know.

☐ **Remind them that what goes online stays online.** Deleting a text, post, photos – or whatever – doesn't mean it is really, truly gone. Inappropriate posts can have unpleasant ways of showing up again – even years later – in surprising ways.

☐ **Protect them from being cyberbullied.** Kids can reduce their risk of being cyberbullied in a variety of ways. To start, teach them to never give out their passwords and to always log out of their accounts if they are away from their screen. Warn them about the dangers of "anonymous" commenting apps that can prove particularly insidious for vulnerable kids. Encourage them to be savvy about what they share with the world. The less content they put out there – especially of a provocative or attention-getting nature – the less likely a target they are.

☐ **And guide them away from being a cyberbully.** Be kind. It's the best policy, so preach it and teach it. Tell them:

- Don't spread untruths

- Don't share potentially embarrassing photos or information about others.

- Don't join in on anything simply because it's what all the other kids are doing.

- Don't respond to anything in the heat of anger. Instead, encourage kids to take the high road, to think before contributing anything on social media, and to report concerns – inappropriate posts, another teen who seems in distress – to a responsible adult.

☐ **Be aware of sexting.** Your kids know all about it, and so should you. Sexting – which may be consensual or non-consensual – is the sending or receiving of sexually explicit pictures, videos, or text messages via smartphone, digital camera, or computer. Most often teens consider it a type of flirting, but the consequences can be significant. In 2017 nearly 15% of teens reported having sent a sext while 27% say they have been the recipient (Madigan, et al, 2018). Then there's sextortion (extortion by threatening the release of naked/sexual pictures or videos).

Bottom line: You do not want this content on any of your family devices. Laws related to sexting in most states are behind the technology, but it is important for parents to know: any type of sexual content involving underage children should be considered child pornography (otherwise known as child sexual abuse material).

☐ **Limit their time.** For any of us, the more time we spend on devices of any kind, the harder it is to disengage and be truly present. There is a real-time, real-people world going on right here, right now. Setting expectations and limits for your kids can help them separate from the online world to be part of what is actually happening right in front of them.

☐ **Put controls on their devices.** You can put controls on computers and cell phones that your kids are using. You can also add an option to see your child's exact location when they are using their cell phone. The Resources list below can help get you started, or go to your cell phone provider for help setting up your options.

As with all things child-rearing, keep the lines of communication open, have ongoing discussions about the risks of being online, share your concerns and make sure your kids know you are always, always available for them.

## AMPLIFY YOUR EFFORTS.

This internet age can be unsettling. As a parent, you may feel out of the loop or even isolated in trying to navigate all the risks of both the "real" and online world and stay on top of what your kids are exposed to.

☐ Talk with other parents! Keep your eyes and ears open about what your kids are up to and be a resource for each other. Don't hesitate to reach out to friends, teachers, or other professionals for advice. You are not alone.

---

# RESOURCES:

Anderson M, Smith A,: *Teens, Social Media & Technology 2018*, May 31, 2018. Pew Research Center. Available at: http://www.pewresearch.org/internet/2018/05/31/teens-social-media-technology-2018/

Fabian-Weber N: 8 Dangers of social media to discuss with kids and teens, 2020. Available at: www.connectsafely.org/tips-to-help-stop-cyberbullying/.

Family Online Safety Institute website: Available at: www.fosi.org/#. (Website).

Hauk C: *How to keep your children safe online: the ultimate guide for the non-Techie parent* 2021. PixelPrivacy. Available at: www.pixelprivacy.com/resources/keep-children-safe-online/

Hendricks D: *Complete history of social media*, 2021 Available at: www.smallbiztrends.com/2013/05/the-complete-history-of-social-media-infographic.html.

HG.org Legal Resources: *What legally makes it child pornography?* Available at: www.hg.org/legal-articles/what-legally-makes-it-child-pornography-38082.

Knorr C: *Parents' Ultimate Guide to Roblox*, 2018. Available at: www.commonsensemedia.org/blog/parents-ultimate-guide-to-roblox-0. (Also in Spanish).

Madigan S, Ly A, Rash CL, et al: *Prevalence of multiple forms of sexting behavior among youth: a systematic review and meta-analysis*. JAMA Pediatrics. 2018;172(4):327–335.

Strasburger VC, Zimmerman H, Temple J, et al: *Teenagers, Sexting, and the Law*. Pediatrics 143,5, May 2019.

Protect Young Eyes website: Available at: http://www.protectyoungeyes.com/. (Website) (Also in many languages)

Symantec: *Parents' best practices to social media security*, 2020. Available at: https://us.norton.com/internetsecurity-kids-safety-stop-stressing-10-internet-safety-rules-to-help-keep-your-family-safe-online.html

# NOTES:

# 36
# Don't Blame THE VICTIM

"There is only one person responsible for child abuse: the perpetrator. When parents bring their children for an abuse/neglect assessment, they are usually asking themselves 'How did this happen?' And they often ask their child questions such as 'Why didn't you tell me?' or 'Didn't you know that was wrong?' The problem is that this approach puts the child in the position of trying to explain what happened and what their role was. They are the victims and should not be asked to explain!"

Discovering that your child has been the victim of abuse is one of the most dreaded parenting scenarios imaginable, and the fallout can be intense. Anger, guilt, fear, sadness, anxiety: these are some of the emotions parents can expect to feel following a revelation of this magnitude. Anger at the perpetrator. Guilt for not preventing it from happening. Sadness at the loss of innocence. Anxiety over what it will all mean. Fear it could happen again – or that life as you know it may change.

It's a *lot* to manage. But the singular, non-negotiable rule in any child abuse situation is this: Never blame the victim.

That may sound simple enough, especially if the alleged perpetrator is not well known to you or if you have always felt like something was "off" about that person. But reality can be complicated. In the all-too-frequent cases where the perpetrator is a family member, a trusted friend, a love interest, or perhaps a relied-upon child care provider, the urge to deflect blame can be intense. Those aforementioned emotions can run away from us, skewing our logic and messing with our brains.

It's easy to understand why. If you blame the alleged perpetrator and that person happens to be a close family member or friend, your family structure, living arrangements, or financial situation may be threatened. Holidays or family gatherings will be different. Relationships with other family members or friends may become strained.

Believing the allegations against a loved one may also make you wonder about your part in all of this. Is it a testament to your parenting abilities? Are you somehow responsible? Will other people think you're a bad caregiver? Blaming or not believing your child in abuse situations can be an attempt to hold onto life as you know it.

Studies show that many children opt not to disclose sexual abuse for fear that they will not be believed – or perhaps even blamed. And, in many cases where abuse *was* reported, but the caregiver failed to respond appropriately, those children harbored feelings of anger and betrayal throughout their adulthood.

Pave the path to healing by striving to be the protector and advocate your child needs you to be.

## CHAMPION THE TRUTH.

It's natural and normal to both want to protect and support your child *and* still have questions. "Why didn't you tell me sooner?" "What were you doing there?" "Why didn't you try to stop it?" can run on an endless loop through your mind. While well-intentioned, questions like these ultimately place blame with the child, feel like interrogation, and can result in additional trauma.

If you suspect that an abusive episode has occurred, here are some suggestions for your approach. (Please note: *if you are just learning that an abusive episode may have occurred, it is extremely important that you **do not** try to get all the details from the child about* *what happened. That is the role of professionals. Your role is just to assure yourself that there is a reason to be suspicious, not to verify that an act has actually occurred.)*

- ☐ Encourage your child to open up by finding a comfortable, safe place to talk.

- ☐ Take what your child says seriously.

- ☐ Acknowledge how difficult it is to share information about the abuse and listen openly without judgment.

- ☐ Avoid a response that displays horror or shock.

- ☐ Reassure your child that they have done nothing wrong.

- ☐ Allow the child to share at their own pace – limiting the number of questions you ask, not making promises and remaining supportive. Ask them: "Has somebody been touching you?" or a similar question. (A somewhat vague question can help you gauge the situation and guide additional questions.) Listen closely, avoid judgment, or blame and be reassuring.

## AMPLIFY YOUR EFFORTS.

If you have suspicions that an abusive or neglectful incident has occurred, call your Child Abuse Hotline (1-800-422-4453) for direction about how to proceed with the information you have. *You do not have to make the case – just report your suspicions.*

- ☐ If you suspect any child is being abused, take action by seeking help. That is your job as a responsible adult.

- ☐ Let the child know you are going to involve others who can help. Before reporting the suspected abuse, let the child know you will be doing so (and be clear you are not asking for their permission).

From a prevention standpoint, tell your children that they should let you know when something doesn't feel "right," along with what worries them about interactions with other children or adults.

# RESOURCES:

Childhelp: *Handling child abuse disclosures.* Available at: www.childhelp. org/wp-content/uploads/2014/10/Disclosure-PDF.pdf.

Feiring C, Taska L, Lewis M: Adjustment following sexual abuse discovery: The role of shame and attributional style. *Developmental Psychology, 38:1: 79-92, 2002.*

Hunter SV: Disclosure of child sexual abuse as a life-long process: Implications for health professionals. *The Australian and New Zealand Journal of Family Therapy, 32:2: 159-172, 2011.*

Rape, Abuse & Incest national Network (RAINN): *Help for parents of children who have been sexually abused by family members.* Available at: www.rainn.org/articles/help-parents-children-who-have-been-sexually-abused-family-members.

RAINN: *If you suspect a child is being harmed.* Available at: www.rainn. org/articles/if-you-suspect-child-being-harmed.

# NOTES:

# 37

# *Be* "TRAUMA INFORMED"

"This is a story I have frequently heard: 'My parents divorced when I was eight years old, and it devastated me. On top of being hurt and angry, for the longest time I thought that it was my fault - that if I had been a better kid, it wouldn't have happened.' It was every cliché you've ever heard of, but for me, it was true, and my parents were were so caught up in their own issues, it took them a long time to really pay attention. Fortunately, they finally realized the impact of everything and helped me through it."

A perfect, pure, brand-new baby is placed in your arms and, just like that, the universe tilts. That's the power of love – and the weight of parental responsibility. In a blink, you know you would do anything to protect this little human.

And you try. You keep them warm and fed. You take them to every well-baby checkup, you use the right kind of car seat, you strap on their helmet when they ride a bicycle. But eventually a time comes when you learn (because you always knew) that it is impossible to protect your children forever. Sometimes, bad things happen to kids and their families.

It could be divorce, the loss of a home, or experiencing or witnessing violence. It could be the death of a parent, friend, or family

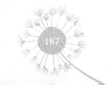

member. It could be abuse or neglect. It's these bigger, life-changing kind of events that are considered to cause "trauma."

Also known as Adverse Childhood Experiences (ACEs), trauma is most harmful to children when it occurs repeatedly or 'piles up.' The brain remembers trauma in special ways. When similar smells, sights, sounds, or thoughts are experienced later, they may trigger the original trauma response. Younger children or children who lack strong social support can be especially vulnerable.

This is where you come in. Children need to be reassured that they are safe and protected from the original bad thing that happened to them. Being a trauma-informed parent simply means that you are aware a child may be hurt – even if they are silent about it – and that you have strategies ready to support them. "Trauma-informed care" is a term used by health care providers. What it really means is they work to provide safe environments for kids and their parents; places where trauma is recognized and care provided to reduce the negative effects it might have. Building resilience is a key goal. Positive childhood experiences and support can lessen the effects of ACEs.

## HELP HEAL THE HURT.

How can you understand what is going through your child's mind, and what can you do about it? First step: tap into your brain's time-machine feature and put yourself in your child's place and age. Just imagine what a negative event might mean to them. They may feel fear, helplessness, or panic. For long-term trauma, such as neglect, they may be worried about having their basic needs met: food, shelter, safety, love.

Sure, not every child will experience a particular event as a trauma. Some may be impacted while others emerge perfectly okay. So, be on the lookout for behaviors that aren't typical. Your child may be quieter or whinier than usual. They may begin wetting the bed again, start having problems in school, or show a lack of motivation. They may feel unsafe or have unexplained outbursts. They may be depressed. The confusion and upset kids experience are often revealed through their bodies, thoughts, emotions, or behaviors.

Now, what can you do?

☐ **Recognize the impact trauma has had on children and advocate for them.** Sometimes those without full knowledge of what a child has experienced will misdiagnose the problem as attention deficit disorder, learning disability, or some other condition. Be sure to tell health care providers about any known traumatic experience(s) so that they can adjust their care accordingly.

☐ **Help them feel safe.** Reassure kids they are not alone and that you and others are there to help and protect them.

☐ **Provide home routines that are predictable.** This helps build trust.

☐ **Let children own and express their feelings.** Equip them with words to describe their feelings and acceptable ways to deal with them, then praise them when they do.

☐ **Help kids hold onto good relationships** that are positive in their lives.

☐ **Seek trauma-informed therapy.** *Don't try to manage a child who has been traumatized by yourself.* It takes time, thought, and skill to help kids cope with and emerge from bad experiences with positive self-esteem and good feelings about their world. Professionals trained to help kids are so important. Be sure to ask the therapist: "Are you familiar with research about the effects of trauma on children?" "What experience do you have working with kids who have experienced trauma?" "How will you determine whether my child's symptoms are related to trauma?" and "How does a trauma history influence your treatment?"

☐ **Help kids understand that sometimes bad things happen to good people,** and that they are still good despite what has happened. The trauma doesn't define them, but is rather just one thing that happened in their life.

☐ **Take care of yourself.** Not only are you caring for a traumatized child, but you may well be coping with that same trauma. Go easy.

## AMPLIFY YOUR EFFORTS.

Foster or adoptive parents can be especially likely to encounter situations with children who have experienced trauma and may benefit from additional help to master trauma-informed parenting skills. Luckily, there are several resources available. Talk with your child's primary care provider or a mental health care specialist to find good, local places to get the support you and your child need.

---

# RESOURCES:

American Academy of Pediatrics and Dave Thomas Foundation for Adoption: *Parenting After Trauma: Understanding Your Child's Needs,* 2013. Available at: www.healthychildren.org/English/family-life/family-dynamics/adoption-and-foster-care/Pages/Parenting-Foster-Adoptive-Children-After-Trauma.aspx

Child Welfare Information Gateway: *Parenting a child who has experienced trauma,* 2014. Available at: www.childwelfare.gov/pubPDFs/child-trauma

Kids Health: *Child abuse.* 2021. Nemours Foundation. Available at: https://kidshealth.org/en/parents/child-abuse.html. (Also in Spanish)

National Child Traumatic Stress Network: *The Essentials of Trauma-informed Parenting.* Available at: www.nctsn.org/trauma-informed-care/trauma-informed-systems/child-welfare/essential-elements

Rosenthal L: *Negative behavior as a form of communication: How to be a trauma-informed parent, 2019.* Available at: https://www.nationwidechildrens.org/family-resources-education/700childrens/2019/08/how-to-be-a-trauma-informed-parent

---

# NOTES:

# 38

## CHOOSE YOUR WORDS *Wisely*

"Even though our intentions may not be malicious, we adults often use certain words out of habit – I hate *that*, this is *stupid*, don't be *dumb*, such a *loser*, etc. Kids are sponges, so it's no surprise that these words quickly transfer to their vocabularies. Such careless comments can even influence self-esteem when children are on the receiving end of them. Not long ago, I learned a valuable lesson from a little friend. At his preschool, it was suggested that rather than saying that he 'hated' something, he could try saying 'it's not my cup of tea.' That stuck with me. Now I often catch myself mid-blurt and try to think about what I really mean—and how those words will be perceived by their recipient—when I'm about to say something like 'that's a dumb idea.' Perhaps 'that's something to consider' or 'I hadn't thought of it that way' is a more respectful – and less judgmental – way to get my point across. Listening to ourselves and considering the words we choose can quickly shift thoughtless communication to thoughtful communication, and set a more positive tone for those little sponges to absorb."

Whoever came up with the line "sticks and stones may break my bones but names will never hurt me" should be called out for failing to check the facts. Words win and lose political elections, have ignited wars and launched love affairs. *Never* underestimate their power.

When it comes to communicating with our kids, well, sometimes the words we hear coming out of our own mouths take us by surprise. Our patience gets tested and we blurt out things we later regret – especially in the heat of the moment.

Here's what we all need to know, though: those moments when we lose it and say the wrong things to our kids may – over time – do as much harm to their minds as any physical object might do to their bodies. Shouting and yelling takes a toll on even the youngest, non-verbal children. It can reinforce withdrawal early on and heighten insecurity in the long run. Verbal abuse—like physical abuse and other traumatic events—can even compromise brain development.

It doesn't take an expert to understand that kids who are verbally humiliated will have self-esteem issues. Children who endure frequent, degrading verbal discipline are also likely to show higher levels of anxiety, depression, anger, and hostility. They can become hyper-sensitive and guilt-ridden. Consequently, they're more likely to engage in aggressive or antisocial behavior, or even abuse drugs. Love and affection are great, but all the hugs in the world won't undo the damage inflicted by verbal attacks.

As might be expected, kids who frequently misbehave tend to experience more harsh verbal discipline than others. But harsh words often perpetuate their acting out, so it becomes a vicious cycle.

## SAY WHAT?

Bottom line: When the urge to lash out strikes, stop and take a breath. Kids seek and need approval from parents and other adults in their world, such as teachers and coaches. When they don't get it, their confidence suffers. By modeling disrespectful language, parents increase the odds their kids will turn into bullies or become depressed, withdrawn, or even self-harmful.

Let's think before we speak. Choose our words wisely. Take deep breaths and make sure we're in control of our own emotions before responding to the actions of our kids.

Here are five simple suggestions for keeping things positive—especially when discipline is involved:

- ☐ **When voicing disapproval, take a second to ask yourself three questions.** Is what you are about to say true? Is it kind? Is it necessary?

- ☐ **Don't compare your kids to others.** On the contrary, reinforce the fact that their gifts (and the gifts of every human being) are unique. Acknowledge, compliment, and cultivate their strengths.

- ☐ **Always try to be warm and responsive.** Look for opportunities to celebrate and praise. Do so genuinely and frequently.

- ☐ **Avoid sarcasm.** Children are "concrete" thinkers and often do not understand sarcasm. They typically take words at their face value.

- ☐ **Don't project your anger with others on your kids.** It's not their fault you had a bad day – or a troubled childhood. Process your challenging emotions with friends and counselors, and save your very best for your kids.

In the end, these are the ways we should talk with *everyone*—not just our kids. But parents matter more to kids than anybody else in their world. Aim to be the person your kids want you to be – from your words to your actions.

## AMPLIFY YOUR EFFORTS.

Words can often be reactive rather than proactive, but you have the power to turn that story around. *This* Monday morning – consider sending your children out the door with these positive ideas dancing in their heads:

"I love you no matter what."

"I'm proud of you."

"You've got this."

"You're such a hard worker."

"How can I help?"

If you hear others speaking in negative terms to kids, let them know that their words are hurtful and need to be changed.

Boost the kids in your domain up. Fill their brains and hearts with kind and supportive words. Tell them you love them, then watch how their worlds expand.

# RESOURCES:

EMC: *The effects of positive words on kids,* 2021. Available at: https://www.engagingmathcircles.com/blog/ the-effects-of-positive-words-on-kids/

Fields RD: *Sticks and stones—hurtful words damage the brain,* October 2010. Available at: http:// psychologytoday.com/us/blog/the-new-brain/201010/ sticks-and-stones-hurtful-words-damage-the-brain

Laungari D: Mind your language: How words can impact your child, 2020. Available at: https://www.resetyoureveryday.com/ mind-your-language-how-words-can-impact-your-child/

University of Pittsburg: *Flying off the handle: cruel words from parents are like 'sticks and stones,'* 2013. Available at: https://www.futurity.org/ cruel-words-parents-just-bad-sticks-stones/

Zolten K, Long N: *Parent/child* communication, 2006. University of Tennessee Center for Effective Parenting. Handouts. Available at: https://parenting-ed.org/wp-content/themes/parenting-ed/files/ handouts/communication-parent-to-child.pdf

# NOTES:

# 39
## DISCIPLINE WITH *Love*

"Disciplining children is not easy! The most challenging part of parenting is understanding your child's developmental stages—and then figuring out the most loving, consistent, and developmentally-appropriate way to discipline them without crossing the line into physical punishment. It's my role as a pediatric professional to help parents along this journey, so that both children and parents can be spared the trauma of physical abuse."

There are many days as a parent when deciding how best to discipline feels like every bit the 10-letter word that it is. Such is the level of frustration, angst, and controversy it stirs up. It's a tricky, touchy subject.

Attitudes and opinions about if, when, why and how to discipline vary from generation to generation and family to family (and sometimes from child to child). Figuring out the best way to react when kids misbehave is, quite possibly, one of the most challenging aspects of parenthood. But if we're serious about building a better world for kids, we need to examine how we help them manage their behavior. And our goal should always be to positively teach good behavior, not just focus on the bad.

Most Americans believe that physical punishment is acceptable—despite compelling evidence to the contrary. Until recently,

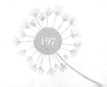

physical punishment was *not* viewed as abuse. But there's been a whole lot of research that increasingly shows such punishment *is* a form of abuse, with significant negative consequences.

While parents who physically punish their kids may sometimes get the immediate results they desire (specifically, compliant children), the practice is ineffective and counter-productive over the long haul. Studies show that physical punishment is harmful to children physically, emotionally, psychologically, and socially. And abuse often leads to more abuse—resulting in an unwanted generational legacy. Kids who comply as a result of physical punishment, or the threat of it, do so out of fear, and fear is a terrible long-term motivator.

According to experts, physical punishment can lead to:

- Increased antisocial behavior and acceptance of violent behavior.
- Higher levels of aggression—toward parents, siblings, peers, and eventual partners
- Poor academic performance
- Compromised family relationships
- Teen delinquency – older kids who fight sometimes get suspended or arrested.
- Depression, anxiety, hopelessness, and other mental health issues
- Substance abuse
- Spousal assault

Prolonged physical or emotional abuse or neglect also likely reduces the brain's grey matter with its many neurons, which compromises a child's ability to learn and can even lower their IQ. There are no known positive effects of physical punishment – and to date, more than 30 countries have banned such punishment, even in the home. Children should never be taught that the strongest can be mean to the younger or less powerful in society.

The bottom line: parents who model aggression are telling children that hurting others is an acceptable way to deal with problems. Given that children learn so much by the example set by adults, it's fair for adults to ask themselves: Is *this* the example we want to set?

## BE YOUR KIDS' BEST TEACHER.

A good place to start is to shift thinking away from "punishment" to instead embrace "discipline." What's the difference? Discipline stems from the word "disciple" or "instructor" – an evolution which places the focus on *teaching* children proper ways to behave. On the flip side, "punishment" implies pain or treating another in an unfair or harsh way – a definition that is associated with retribution and fear.

The temperament and developmental stages of children are cues to understanding how to best discipline them. To help children become more responsible and caring through adolescence and into adulthood, there *are* effective ways to respond to misbehavior without resorting to physical punishment. Here are ten guiding principles:

☐ **Treat children the way *you* would like to be treated.**

☐ **Be empathetic – kids have feelings, too!**

☐ **Let the little things go; ignoring attention-seeking misbehavior can be more effective than punishing it.**

☐ **Give both your child and yourself a "time out" during difficult interactions; look for "win-win" solutions.**

☐ **When arguments get loud, lower your voice.**

☐ **Give your children time to process things.**

☐ **Be realistic about both the discipline you choose and your ability to follow through with it. Aim for natural consequences.**

☐ **Set reasonable boundaries and expectations for behavior (especially in public)—and follow through on consequences** when children misbehave; don't be afraid to leave a store or restaurant, or skip an important event if necessary. Kids learn quickly that you mean business!

☐ **Don't hesitate to negotiate, especially with older children; that helps them understand limits and encourages self-control.**

☐ **Look for opportunities to praise and reward positive behavior.**

The trick for parents is to discipline in ways that positively shape kids' behavior without trespassing into the land of "I crossed the line." Vow to be the best, wisest *teacher* you can be.

## AMPLIFY YOUR EFFORTS.

Effective discipline requires extraordinary patience—and even the most skilled parents sometimes fall short. That's okay. Don't be afraid to ask for help—from other parents, from your pediatrician, or from other health professionals. Besides individual counseling, parenting support groups or parenting classes can be very helpful in learning new coping skills and allowing you to feel less alone in your frustration.

And when the going gets tough, remember to just breathe!

## RESOURCES:

Akitunde T: *Why Black people should stop spanking their kids*. Matermea. Available at: https://matermea.com/does-corporal-punishment-have-a-place-in-the-black-community/

American Psychological Association: *ACT/Parents Raising Safe Kids*. Available at: http://www.apa.org/act/

Case H: *The long-term effects of physical punishment on a child*, 2018. Available at: www.livestrong.com/article/213859-long-term-effects-of-physical-punishment-on-a-child/.

Castelloe MS: *How spanking harms the brain: why spanking should be outlawed*, 2012. Available at: https://psychologytoday.com/us/blog/the-me-in-we/201202/how-spanking-harms-the-brain.

Durrant J, Ensom R: *Physical punishment of children: lessons from 20 years of research*, 2012. Available at: http://www.ncbi.nlm.nih.gov/pmc/articles/PMC3447048.

Hunt J: *22 alternatives to punishment*, 2013. Available at: www.naturalchild.org/jan_hunt/22_alternatives.html

Klika B, Merrick M: *Physical punishment: Attitudes, behaviors, and norms associated with its use across the US*, 2020. Prevent Child Abuse America. Available at: https://www.preventchildabuse.org/resources/physical-punishment-attitudes-behaviors-and-norms-associated-with-its-use-across-the-us.

# NOTES:

# 40
# *Keep* YOUR COOL

Its 5:00 p.m., I'm exhausted and so are my kids. Dinner is far from ready, Mom will be late coming home and on top of that, the car is making a suspicious new rattling noise. At that precise moment, my 12 year son announces: 'I forgot my homework. We need to go back to school and get it.' to which I instantly fire back: 'Not again! The school is closed. This is the fifth time this term that you forgot your school work and we promised your teacher we wouldn't let that happen again!' His response: 'It's your fault. You rushed me to leave on time so I forgot!". I quickly reach my boiling point and just want to scream. I've lost my cool."

Oh, how sweet it would be to – *just once* – throw a tantrum with the reckless abandon of a two-year-old. To just full-on lay it all out there: screaming, foot-stomping, floor-writhing, name-calling. The whole nine yards.

Alas, we are adults and that type of behavior just doesn't fly. But children communicate their needs in the most effective ways they know how – ways that don't always match up with what we would prefer. Sometimes, unpleasant behavior is just their way of communicating. For the toddler and preschool set, they are just learning what hot buttons are all about – behaviors that get attention but make others mad and may not get the desired outcome.

Their intentions are not to be hurtful but simply to get attention for something they want or to express an emotion they are feeling.

Regardless, only the most calm, cool and skilled among us manage to never fall into the kid-powered tantrum trap. Many parents are skilled at controlling their emotions most of the time, some have trouble occasionally, and others have chronic challenges keeping a lid on their temper.

Obviously, we want to set a good example for our children and maintaining our cool when the heat is on is a big part of that. Kids mirror and learn from us. Very often, the behavior we see in them is a direct reflection of what they see in us. The two best reasons to learn how to handle your anger?

1. Your kids are watching.
2. You don't want to hurt your kids physically or emotionally.

## KEEP CALM AND PARENT ON.

Let's get this out there: anger is normal. It can even be constructive. It's all a matter of what you choose to do with it. And it is a choice. So how can you work to turn your temper in a positive direction?

☐ **Remind yourself that you are your child's helper and teacher.** Discipline yourself. Your child may not have intended to get you riled, but they did. Your reaction to these moments impacts them. Your calm, measured response is a powerful teaching moment.

☐ **Don't take it personally.** Your kids' behavior is not a reflection of your worth and rarely of your skills as a parent. If your child misbehaves in public, the reactions of others matter little (and most critics are unlikely to have been parents anytime in the recent past anyway). What matters is that you take care of the situation effectively.

☐ **Know your triggers.** Jot down some common scenarios that cause you to blow up at your kids. What situations or events do you know make you mad, stressed or put you on edge? Identifying your triggers leads you to understand yourself better, which can help end the anger cycle by bringing awareness to your response.

☐ **Decide what you are going to do ahead of time**. Once you understand what situations cause you stress or lead you to become angry, you're in a better position to plan ahead. For instance, if carpool sibling squabbling makes you see red, make it clear to your children what the consequences of misbehavior will be.

☐ **Delay your reaction.** Your child threw a toy car at point-blank range and broke a lamp. You're fuming. The first thing you should do is...nothing. Waiting even a few seconds helps the hot flame of anger start to sputter, placing you in a much more level-headed position to deal with the situation. If your anger level remains close to the boiling point, excuse yourself. Go into another room and take some deep breaths until you begin to feel calmer.

☐ **Be prepared to apologize.** If you lose your temper, admit it to your child, but not overly emotionally. If you need to apologize, do it simply: "I'm sorry I yelled at you, sweetie. Sometimes grown-ups lose their tempers too. I'm working on it." Have a support person that you can talk to later about those situations when you feel you have lost control. Verbalizing your feelings helps with processing and awareness.

☐ **If you must, throw a tantrum.** Just don't do it in front of your kids. Instead, do something physical, like push-ups or jumping jacks. Leave the room to catch your breath if you have to. If you can go to a gym or take a walk, go! Direct your frustrations at the pavement on a run or explaining what happened to a confidant.

☐ **Give yourself a break.** We all have tough moments and difficult days. Show yourself compassion, and show some to others as well.

## AMPLIFY YOUR EFFORTS.

If for you losing your temper leads to physical violence or verbal abuse, get help now! Take responsibility and don't feel ashamed or afraid. One immediate place to get help is through the Child Abuse Hotlines available in every state. The 24-hour National Hotline at 1-800-422-4453 can put you in touch with local providers of child abuse services.

Proper support from a trained professional can help you unravel the story behind your own reactions and behavior, and equip you with new coping skills. That is bound to boost your relationship with your kids – and very likely other important relationships in your life – and help set a new direction for generations to come.

---

# RESOURCES:

Eanes R: *8 ways to keep your cool when you're about to blow up on your kids*, 2018. Available at: www.workingmother.com/8-ways-to-keep-your-cool-when-youre-about-to-blow-up-on-your-kids#page-3.

Lascala M: *How to keep your cool around your kids when you're ready to blow*, 2019. Available at: http://www.goodhousekeeping.com/life/parenting/a28719940/keep-your-cool-with-kids/.

Lehman J: *Temper, temper: keeping your cool when kids push your buttons* ,2018. Available at: www.empoweringparents.com/article/temper-temper-keeping-your-cool-when-kids-push-your-buttons/.

The Center for Parenting Education: *Parents Anger: Turning down the heat in your home*. Available at: www.centerforparentingeducation.org/library-of-articles/anger-and-violence/parents-anger-turning-down-the-heat-in-your-home/.

# NOTES:

# 41
## PUT GUNS BEHIND *Locks*

> "Keeping kids safe around guns requires everyone's involvement—no matter where you sit on the political fence. While people's attitudes about guns may differ around the country, few will dispute that safety is the most important factor. Gun safety should be taught to all children—just like we teach them not to get into a car with a stranger. It's that simple."

This isn't about politics. This is about our kids and gun safety, and facts are facts:

- 1 in 4 Americans live in a home with a gun (Pew Research, 2021) and 1 in 3 homes with children in America have guns.
- Gun injuries are now the leading cause of death for children of all ages in the U.S. – surpassing motor vehicle accidents and other causes of injury (Schaeffer, 2021).
- 1.7 million kids live in a home with unlocked, loaded guns, and 40% of those kids know where the gun is stored, though the majority of parents do not think the children know. Thirty percent of those kids say they have handled the gun.
- People under age 25 – and adolescents in particular – are the most vulnerable to accidental shootings due to

factors including impulsivity, feelings of invincibility and plain old curiosity.

- More than 80% of guns used by youth in suicide attempts were kept in the home of the victim, a relative, or a friend.
- Family conflict, multi-victim events, crime and violence, and firearm suicides are the most common factors for gun violence fatalities in children. Unintentional causes of firearm deaths among children are most commonly related to kids playing with a gun (Fowler, et al, 2017).

All of which leads to one potentially life-or-death question: At this very moment, what stands between your child and access to a gun? Is it a neighbor's front door? Perhaps a couple of walls within your own home? Do you have any idea whether your children's friends have guns in their homes?

Information is power. Know the risks your kids face and then aim to lower them.

## THE LOWDOWN ON LOCKING DOWN.

There are some obvious ways to reduce the chances of a child or adult being harmed by a firearm. So please, take steps today to ensure you or your child is not left holding a smoking gun.

☐ **Lock guns in a secure location** – such as a gun safe, or at minimum with a trigger lock – and keep keys stored in a place inaccessible to children. If you are a non-gun owner who lives with a gun owner, make certain you are fully knowledgeable about the location and storage of both guns and ammunition within your household.

☐ **Keep guns unloaded and separated from ammunition,** which should always be stored in a locked location. Always.

☐ **Treat any gun as if it is loaded**: pointed away from others and keeping fingers off the trigger.

☐ **Don't be shy! Find out if your kids' friends have guns in their homes** – and confirm they are safely stored and locked. If not, invite them to hang out at your house. Don't be afraid to simply ask: "Is there an unlocked gun in your home?"

☐ **Teach children not to touch a firearm should they find one unattended in their home or elsewhere, and to alert an adult.**

## AMPLIFY YOUR EFFORTS.

Consider taking a hunter/gun safety course – and signing your children up for one if your family owns guns or enjoys hunting or shooting hobbies.

Should a young person in your home demonstrate one of the following risk factors: ADHD, family violence, depression, suicide ideation, alcohol or drug abuse, or bullying, you need to take extra precautions regarding firearm safety.

## RESOURCES:

Brady Campaign: *End Family Fire*. Available at: www.bradycampaign. org/gun-violence/topics/children-and-gun-violence.

Children's Hospital of Philadelphia, Center for Injury Research and Prevention: *Gun violence: Facts and statistics*, 2020. Available at: https://violence.chop.edu/gun-vioence-facts-and-statistics

Fowler K, Dahlberg L, Kaileysus T, et al: *Childhood firearm injuries in the United States*, June, 2017. Available at: https://pubmed.ncbi.nlm. nih.gov/28630118

Schaechter S: *Guns in the home*. Healthychildren.org, 2021. Available at: https://www.healthychildren.org/English/safety-prevention/ at-home/Pages/Handguns-in-the-home.aspx

Schaeffer K: *Key facts about Americans and guns*, 2021. Pew
Research Center. Available at: www.pewresearch.org/
fact-tank/2021/09/13/key-facts-about-americans-and-guns/

---

# NOTES:

# PART FOUR

## SOCIAL *Support*

Social support is the provision of assistance or comfort to others, typically to help them cope with biological, psychological, and social stressors. Support may arise from any interpersonal relationship in an individual's social network, involving family members, neighbors, religious institutions, colleagues, caregivers, community agencies, or support groups. It may take the form of tangible help such as helping with chores, providing financial assistance, or giving emotional support that allows the individual to feel valued, accepted and understood.[*]

---

[*]   American Psychological Association

In healthy families, people care for one another. They show love and respect, laugh, have fun and spend time together. There is a real sense of belonging, with friends and extended family who they can count on if they're in need. Outside of the family, developing a solid social network takes time and effort. It may mean becoming active in civic events and projects to make connections. On a broader social support level, there are many service organizations and agencies dedicated to helping families stay well by addressing physical, housing, employment, and other needs. Caring adults outside of the family can serve as role models and mentors, while communities and schools can provide environments where families will feel cared for and cared about.

Families can be prepared to take the first steps to obtain the supportive services they need. The Tips in this section focus on just that, offering suggestions to help you grow and strengthen your social network. Those efforts involve both giving and receiving activities. We didn't coin this, but it's true: *It takes a village to raise a child.*

# 42

# *Build* A SUPPORT NETWORK

"I have moved many times. Each time has been an opportunity
to build a new community for my family, but it is not always
easy! I have learned to be intentional about meeting people.
I take my kids to museums or to story time at the bookstore
or library (some of my closest friends have been made in the
stacks). I scour local online papers and community boards for
opportunities to meet new people, like community gatherings,
classes, concerts or theater productions. A realtor once gave
me phone numbers of other moms in a new area, and although
it was terrifying to call someone I had never met, it was the
best chance I ever took! By being vulnerable and reaching out
to others, I gave my kids and myself the gift of some amazing
friendships and memories that will last a lifetime."

There's a particular kind of irony that comes with parenting young
children: as your family expands, it can feel as if the rest of your
world contracts. Suddenly, you're hunkered down on diaper and
formula duty instead of meeting up with friends for happy hour.
Exhaustion reigns; you're awake at 3 a.m. and nodding off at 5 p.m.
You might feel frustrated, overwhelmed, or painfully bored.

And if you're feeling alone, you're not alone! Loneliness, in fact,
is one of the most common struggles of parenthood and can be felt
even more acutely by new parents, single parents or those who are

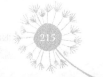

new to a community. Building a strong support network of people you can count on for emotional support, friendship – and sometimes even kid-sitting is key.

Parents who build strong social connections and relationships may also be helping keep their kids safer. Research shows that isolated parents are at higher risk for maltreating their children. Social networking is the best way to combat feelings of isolation, encourage happiness and make us more resilient – all things that help make for better, more well-rounded caregivers.

## BUILD YOURSELF A VILLAGE.

If you are fortunate enough to already have a network of friends or relatives who are a) nearby and b) people you can truly rely on, that's excellent. But if you're new to an area or just don't know many other parents of young kids, you'll need to take extra steps to bust out of the parental isolation zone and meet your people. Test out a few of these oldie-but-goodie tactics.

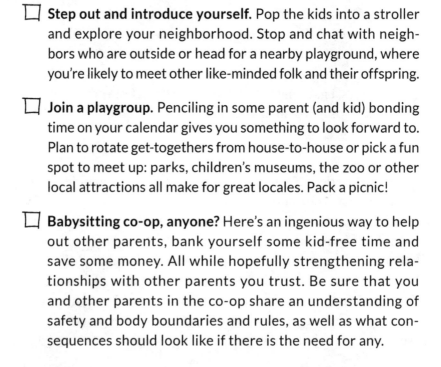

☐ **Step out and introduce yourself.** Pop the kids into a stroller and explore your neighborhood. Stop and chat with neighbors who are outside or head for a nearby playground, where you're likely to meet other like-minded folk and their offspring.

☐ **Join a playgroup.** Penciling in some parent (and kid) bonding time on your calendar gives you something to look forward to. Plan to rotate get-togethers from house-to-house or pick a fun spot to meet up: parks, children's museums, the zoo or other local attractions all make for great locales. Pack a picnic!

☐ **Babysitting co-op, anyone?** Here's an ingenious way to help out other parents, bank yourself some kid-free time and save some money. All while hopefully strengthening relationships with other parents you trust. Be sure that you and other parents in the co-op share an understanding of safety and body boundaries and rules, as well as what consequences should look like if there is the need for any.

☐ **Host a party.** Any kind of party. Craft-making, movie-watching, game-playing, food-eating, whatever. The important thing is to create a time and place to bring together new and old friends, make some memories and forge the kind of friendships you can count on when you need them.

☐ **Head to the library.** Especially for library story time, where all the cool parents and kids are! Introduce yourself to another parent or two. Maybe go for coffee afterwards?

☐ **Sign up for a class.** Check out your local parks and recreation department (if your town has one) or community center for inspiration. Most communities offer activities where parents and kids can participate together, and you're likely to meet *other* parents and kids.

☐ **Welcome others into your circle.** Always, always strive to be the one who spots the new person, the lonely person, the person looking to make a connection – and invite them in. It's just good karma.

☐ **Consider getting involved in a faith-based organization that offers a children's group.**

## AMPLIFY YOUR EFFORTS.

While you're busy building a new support network, help your kids do the same. Research shows that kids who grow up with strong connections and solid friendships are better communicators, more empathetic and end up as happier adults. Suggest they join a friend at a movie or other activity or have them over to play for the afternoon for the afternoon. Invite their mom or dad in for coffee at the same time.

Ask your kids to tell you who they would feel comfortable going to for help or support if needed. Then make sure your kids have contact information for that person (or persons). Be sure to vet those resources for safety and let them know they were selected by your family as a safe person for help if needed. if they need it. Be sure they have their contact information and that they have been vetted for safety.

Work to make your home a welcoming place where your children – and other people's children – want to be. And get to know your kids' friends! As they grow, it will be important for their entire network of friends to know that you're paying attention, you care about them and you're an adult they can trust and count on.

## RESOURCES:

Abrams A: *How to build a successful babysitting cooperative.* 2016. Available at: www.parents.com/baby/childcare/babysitter/ how-to-build-a-successful-babysitting-cooperative/.

Child Welfare Information Gateway: *Social Connections* website. Available at: www.childwelfare.gov/topics/preventing/promoting/ protectfactors/social-connect/.

Children's Bureau: *Social Connection on Child Development* website. Available at: www.all4kids.org/ social-connection-on-child-development/.

Raisingchildren.net.au: *Services and support: an overview.* Available at: https://raisingchildren.net.au/grown-ups/services-support/ about-services-support/services-support

Springer A: *How socially connected are you?* Sept. 5, 2017. Available at: http://www.greatergood.berkeley.edu/article/item/ how_socially_connected_are_you.

Suttie J: *Four ways social support makes you more resilient*, Nov 13, 2017. Available at: www.greatergood.berkeley.edu/article/item/ four_ways_social_support_makes_you_more_resilient.

# NOTES:

# 43

## *Get* THEIR CHECKUPS

"I remember being a new parent and feeling so unsure of what I was doing to care for my new baby. Yes, I knew the basics but it all still felt so strange and I was sometimes overwhelmed with exhaustion and the never-ending vigilance that caring for a child required. My husband took over when he could and was supportive – but I still felt at my wits' end sometimes. One person who always made me feel better was our pediatrician. As I look back, she was the person who always told me I was doing a good job! I needed that feedback and little pat on the back. She was also a person I felt I could talk to if needed. I recommend that you look for a primary care provider (pediatrician or pediatric nurse practitioner) who gives you that pat on the back and can be a resource if you are unsure or need advice."

Middle-of-the-night fevers, playground mishaps, well-baby checkups, *another* ear infection. Does it sometimes feel like you and your pediatric health care provider are spending far too much time together?

If it does, consider yourself fortunate. That means you have access to health care which many families and children do not have. If you don't have health insurance or other financial resources, be sure to turn to your county health department.

Finding a health care provider you respect, trust, and can turn to for advice on matters big and small is a privilege. It also is a powerful strategy for raising healthy kids. The American Academy of Pediatrics recommends that you meet face-to-face with your baby's primary care provider about eight times in your baby's first year alone. The first two years of a child's development are crucial, so they want to see your children regularly to monitor their progress, get them started on their immunization schedule and be able to identify any problems that may arise.

Pediatric physicians and nurse practitioners are trained to support families in broad ways. When you take your child in for a checkup, here's what you can and should expect your provider to do:

- Monitor your child's overall health, including private parts checks for younger kids.
- Explain your child's growth and development in ways you understand.
- Diagnose and treat illnesses – and explain what they are doing and why.
- Provide information on how to prevent injuries and keep your child safe.
- Assist with finding specialists for problems outside their area of expertise.
- Help you with developmental and behavioral issues, or know who to call if your questions are outside their practice comfort zone.

Building a partnership with your health care provider is a two-way street. When you're an active participant in the process, your kids reap the benefits.

## KEEP THEM WELL.

A few tips to help your office visits be as productive as you and your provider want them to be:

☐ **Write down questions** before the visit so you don't forget something important.

☐ **Share *all* the symptoms when there is a concern**, even if you are not asked specifically. Report what you have already done to try to fix the problem and how it worked. The more information you give, the better decisions your provider can make.

☐ **Try to be informed, but don't let information overwhelm you.** The Internet is a great resource, but it can also be a big source of confusion. Talk with your provider about what you have learned and bring printed material if it is helpful to you.

☐ **Stay focused during your visit.** If you can, leave other kids at home, turn off your cell phone, and minimize distractions.

☐ **Use your visit for the problem at hand.** It often just doesn't work well to delve into a significant behavioral problem during, say, a sick-child visit. You might ask, "Do you have the time today to talk with me about a school problem, too?" Schedule a separate visit if needed.

☐ **Take notes.** If there are follow-up activities for you – lab, imaging, pharmacy, another appointment, make a list so you don't miss a step.

☐ **Make the most of other provider resources.** For non-urgent problems, there may be someone else in the office you can talk to. Many practices have nurse practitioners or other professionals who can help with a variety of problems – either over the phone or through an office visit.

☐ **Use electronic medical record resources** if your practice has them available. Email communication, access to the latest test results, visit summaries, scheduling appointments, and other options can make health care more efficient for everyone.

☐ **Give your provider feedback** about what is working or not working for you. Providers need that to improve their work.

And let's not forget the child! Doctor's visits aren't every kid's favorite, but there are a few things you can try to make the experience as positive as possible.

☐ **For younger children**, attempt to schedule the visit at a time when he or she is usually awake and happy. It doesn't always work out, but it's a good place to start! Bringing along things that soothe your child – a toy, book, snack, or blanket – can help de-escalate a child's stress.

☐ **For older kids** who remember previous visits, go through the "script" for the visit so the child knows what to expect. If this visit will be different from previous ones – for instance, they had immunizations last time, but won't this time – let the child know. It may go the other way too, so prepare kids for the difficult points of the visit. Bottom line: Minimize surprises!

☐ **Teens** should be prepared for a visit by themselves. You will likely be asked to wait outside the exam room at least for part of the visit, and that might feel uncomfortable. Remember that this is part of your teen's growing independence and need for privacy. They need to learn to communicate and advocate for themselves. The doctor's office should be a safe place to do just that. The office should give you an opportunity to share your concerns so you won't be entirely left out of the caregiving situation.

## AMPLIFY YOUR EFFORTS.

Please don't limit the scope of health care you seek to a pediatric medical provider. It's vital that kids get regular dental exams, have their eyes checked, and have any mental health or behavioral issues addressed promptly by trained professionals. (Note: The pediatrician's office should conduct eye screenings, but a visit to an optometrist or ophthalmologist is worth considering – especially if you suspect an issue or have a family history of needing corrective lenses or other eye issues.)

Following the doctor's visit tips shared above translates just as well to working with other health professionals. Your commitment to seeking preventive care and staying on top of any issues that arise is not only a gift to your child and family, but to the entire community. Thanks for working to keep everyone healthy!

# RESOURCES:

Canadian Paediatric Society: You and your child's doctor. *Paediatrics & Child Health,* May-June 14(5): 333-334, 2009. Available at http://www.ncbi.nlm.nih.gov/pmc/articles/PMC2706637.

Kids Health: *What's a Nurse Practitioner?* 2015. Available at: http://www.kidshealth.org/en/parents/nurse-practitioner.html.

Kids Health: *Talking to Your Child's Doctor,* 2017. Available at: http://www.kidshealth.org/en/parents/talk-doctor.html.

Kids Health: *Going to the Doctor,* 2017. Available at http://www.kidshealth.org/en/kids/going-to-dr.html.

# NOTES:

# 44

# Celebrate OUR DIFFERENCES!

"One of my favorite books as a kid was called 'Children Just Like Me.' It showed pictures of kids from cultures and countries all over the world. I was transfixed! These kids were my age, they did the same things I did and they liked the same things – playing games with friends, eating snacks, exploring outside. We weren't so different! It was so exciting to learn about their backgrounds. I can still remember that feeling of, 'Oh my goodness—there's a whole wide world out there!'"

Life on this big, round rock we occupy together would be such an utter snooze fest if we were all exactly the same. Truly, so painfully boring.

Yet, wars are waged, walls are built, and people are hurt and even killed over what we think sets us apart. Religion, skin color, language, political beliefs, culture, sexual orientation, gender, age, body type. There's literally no end to the list of traits that distinguish people—because no two of us are the same. So what if – instead of reinforcing what divides us – we were to approach our differences as a bridge to uniting and inspiring us?

Kids are adults-in-training. What we do and say, they mimic. And, curious little sponges that they are, they are professionals at zooming in on differences – and pointing them out. Kids *notice* things, and they want answers.

It is essential that we carefully craft our responses and the messages we give our children if we want to build empathy and tolerance. And why wouldn't we want that? What if we regularly focused on exploring what unites us?

We're all familiar with the expression "fear of the unknown". What we don't know or understand can cause hesitation, suspicion, and separation from others. Educating ourselves, and in turn our children, can lead us to a clearer understanding of why people look the way they look, behave the way they behave, and believe what they believe.

There is a whole, wide world of fascinating people right outside our doors. Let's meet them!

## OPEN THEIR HEARTS.

Nurturing open minds starts at home – and often, in public. Consider incorporating some, or all, of these ideas to widen your child's sense of the world.

- ☐ **Don't shame kids** for their natural questions about human differences. Kids want to make sense of their world. Wanting to place similar things in patterned "boxes" is normal. Instead of saying, "Don't ask those questions!" try something like, "Because we're all different! See how I have long hair and you have short hair?"

- ☐ **Teach them** words or phrases in different languages to spark curiosity and joy: Te quiero = I love you!

- ☐ **Encourage** kids to make and eat foods from different countries.

- ☐ **Explore museums** to learn about ancient civilizations and the history that ties us together. Help kids discover that it really is a small world, after all.

- ☐ **Attend local cultural festivals** where the whole family can discover the dress, dance, food and customs of another country.

☐ **Take a day trip** to a neighborhood or town known for a different ethnicity. Explore the restaurants and stores there.

☐ **Consider attending religious services for a different faith,** especially if you have someone who can explain what is happening during the service.

Most important, learn to talk with people and be open to their stories. There is so much to learn – and everyone's history is interesting when you dive deep enough!

## AMPLIFY YOUR EFFORTS.

☐ **Learn more about your own family's history**. Consider signing up for Ancestry.com, 23andMe or another service to explore your roots. What an eye opener that can be!

☐ **Spearhead a multicultural "festival" at your kids' school where students are encouraged to share their family and cultural traditions.**

☐ **If you have a travel bug and are fortunate enough to be able to indulge it, go crazy**! Soak in the sights, smells, sounds and tastes of a different country or even city! You don't have to go international to experience something new. Shop in the local grocery stores, visit temples or cathedrals. Talk to the locals and encourage your kids to ask questions.

## RESOURCES:

AllDayMonkey: *7 challenges faced by multicultural families (and why they can be advantages)*. Available at: www.momentsaday.com/7-challenges-faced-multicultural-families/.

Alwine R: *10 Ways to keep your adopted child's cultural connection*. Empowering Solo Moms Everywhere. Available at: https://esme.com/resources/adoption/help-your-adopted-child- maintain-a-cultural-connection

Chrissy: *How to teach your child about different cultures: 11 fun ways*, 2021. Available at: www.funlovingfamilies.com/how-to-teach-your-child-about-different-cultures/

Epstein E: Parenting kids in a multicultural family. LA Parent, June 7, 2015. Available at: www.laparent.com/parenting-kids-in-a-multicultural-family/.

Families embracing diversity: *The best tips for raising multicultural children*, 2019. Available at: http://www.familiesembracingdiversity.com/best-tips-raising-multicultural-child/.

Honey M: *Incorporating LGBTQIA + Content in History Lessons*. June 14, 2019. George Lucas Educational Foundation. Edutopia. Available at: www.edutopia.org/article/incorporating-lgbtqia-content-history-lessons.

Spicer S: *Teach your kids about different cultures*. Today's Parent. July 5, 2010. Available at: www.todaysparent.com/family/teach-your-kids-about-different-cultures/.

Teaching Tolerance: *Culture in the Classroom*. Available at: http://www.tolerance.org/culture-classroom

Tirrell-Corbin C: *How to teach children about cultural awareness and diversity*, August 4, 2015. PBS for Parents. Available at: https://www.pbs.org/parents/thrive/how-to-teach-children-about-cultural-awareness-and-diversity

Van Heusden B: *Education Talks: Why Cultural Education Matters*, April 29, 2016.

# NOTES:

# 45

## *Transcend* GENDER

"When my son was three years old, he asked for a Barbie for his birthday. He specifically requested a Scuba Barbie because he wanted to let her swim in the tub during his bath time. I braced myself for the objection I expected from his dad but to my surprise and delight, he was quite supportive of the Barbie purchase. From that day on, we never worried about whether toys were intended for girls or boys. We acquired the Barbie and several other 'non-stereotypical' toys for Sean over the years. We were led by his interests and desires and encouraged him to explore and experiment. Sean grew up knowing that his mom could not only cook and clean, but also mow the lawn, assemble furniture, and repair the plumbing. Sean is now the father of a little girl, and I am a grandmother for the first time. I'm looking forward to exploring and encouraging my granddaughter's interests, whatever they may be!"

"*So, what are you having? A girl or a boy?!*"

That is *the* question; the one that 100% (ballpark guess) of expectant parents hear, endlessly, from friends, family and total strangers. The answer – girl or boy – matters to us because it informs our perceptions and expectations for pretty much everything, from the color of the nursery we decorate to the toys we purchase to clothing, hairstyle, academics, sports, behavioral and career expectations. Girls do this. Boys do that. Simple, right?

Not really. Sexuality, sexual orientation, gender identity, gender roles. These are terms we now hear almost every day, which is a huge change from even a few years ago. They each mean something different and, yes, it can be confusing. So let's break down their meanings:

*Sexuality* can be defined as the way a person experiences and expresses themselves sexually. This can carry over into a person's biologic, erotic, physical, emotional, social or even spiritual feelings and behaviors.

*Sexual orientation* relates to a person's sexual interest in another person. This is where terms like homosexual, heterosexual or bisexual – to name a few – come into play. Sexual orientation typically emerges in adolescence, when teens begin to consider whether they are more attracted sexually to people of their own sex, the opposite sex, both, or none. It is not something that can be changed by parenting style.

*Gender identity* is an individual's perception of being a particular gender which may or may not correspond with their birth sex.

*Gender roles* are the characteristics, behaviors, dress and/or mannerisms that society associates as belonging to either men or women (or boys or girls) – and they have changed over time. Eighty years ago, women were expected to stay home, raise the kids and take care of the house. Today, both men and women are free to work outside the home or stay home with the kids. Boys and girls can play with dolls or toy trucks, have long or short hair, or wear whatever color they choose. Just as a child's personality emerges over time, gender expression may develop and reveal itself in stages over a period of years.

By now we've all learned, through increased social awareness, that gender identity isn't always clearly defined. Not everyone fits neatly into their expected gender "box." The human development timeline suggests that, around the age of two to three years, kids become aware of the differences between boys and girls, and will identify themselves as one or the other. For some, gender identity remains fluid and may shift over time.

For most children, their assigned gender (what we understand each person's gender to be at birth) and gender identity are aligned. But for some, the reality is more complex. What causes an individual to differ from their assigned gender is a complicated and hard-to-understand process, rooted in a combination of biology, development, socialization, and culture.

Evidence suggests that childhood trauma is not a factor in gender identity development, nor is parenting style. A child also cannot become transgender as a result of peer pressure, and their gender identity cannot be changed through interventions. Understanding and accepting our children – especially when who they are is different from our original expectations – is one of parenting's biggest challenges. But *you* are your child's champion and advocate, and the way you choose to respond to and parent a transgender child will reverberate throughout their life.

## OPEN YOUR MIND – AND YOUR HEART.

Let your child's development unfold naturally by opening their world. Let them play with Barbies and toy trucks, climb trees and dress up in costumes – regardless of gender. Read them books that celebrate the fact that anyone can be a nurse or electrician or teacher or senator – and it's all okay! Show all your kids how to wash dishes, vacuum the house and change a tire. By doing so, you perform a vital community service.

If, as your child grows, it becomes evident their sexual orientation or gender identity is not what you expected or first imagined, remember, your number one job is to love them no matter what. Whether you recognized your child was transgender in early childhood, or they reveal their identity or sexual orientation in their teen years or later, they need you to love them and support them for who they are.

Bullying and discrimination are real. And few groups are more bullied and less understood than our LGBTQ community and children who express their gender roles differently. This isolation can lead to mental health crises that can be life-threatening. Studies have revealed that more than half of transgender teens who identify as male and 30 percent who identify as female have attempted suicide.

Be prepared to advocate for your child – with schools, friends, family, medical professionals, whomever, and prioritize making your home a welcoming, safe place for every family member. And teach your children to accept their classmates and others in the community who identify as LGBTQ+. Having even one accepting friend can change a life and help lead to positive changes in the community – ultimately protecting all children and their families.

## AMPLIFY YOUR EFFORTS.

Gender identity and sexual orientation are complex issues with huge social and psychological implications we can't begin to fully address in this book. For more guidance, support and information, please contact your family's physician for resources in your area. Focus on getting and keeping yourself – and your child – equipped to manage this and many life challenges.

---

# RESOURCES:

Duron L: 7 books that teach kids about the fluidity of gender and the importance of acceptance. Available at: https://www.readbrightly. com/8-books-that-teach-kids-about-the-fluidity-of-gender-and-the-importance-of-acceptance/

Childwelfare Information Gateway: *Resources for families of LGBTQ+ Youth*. Available at: www.childwelfare.gov/topics/systemwide/diverse-populations/lgbtq/lgbt-families

Hassanein R: *New Study reveals shocking rates of attempted suicide among transgender adolescents*, 2018. Available at: https://www.hrc.org/news/new-study-reveals-shocking-rates-of-attempted-suicide-among-trans-adolescents

Head Start/ECLKC. National Center on Parent, Family and Community Engagement: *Healthy gender development and young children: a guide for early childhood programs and professionals*, 2021. Available at: https://www.eclkc.ohs.acf.hhs.gov/publication/healthy-gender-development-young-children

Rafferty J: *Gender identity development in children*, 2018. Healthy Children.org. Available at: https://www.healthychildren.org/English/ages-stages/gradeschool/Pages/Gender-Identity-and-Gender-Confusion-In-Children.aspx (Available in Spanish)

Rafferty J: *Gender-diverse and transgender children*, 2018. Healthy Children.org. Available at: https://www.healthychildren.org/English/ages-stages/gradeschool/Pages/Gender-Diverse-Transgender-Children.aspx (Available in Spanish)

Rafferty J: *Parenting a gender-diverse child: hard questions answered*, 2018. Available at: https://www.healthychildren.org/English/ages-stages/gradeschool/Pages/Parenting-a-Gender-Diverse-Child-Hard-Questions-Answered.aspx (Available in Spanish).

Welcoming Schools: *Great diverse children's books with transgender, non-binary and gender expansive children*. (See website for lists)

---

# NOTES:

# 46

## BE A *Mentor*

> "I used to work as a nanny for four-year-old twin girls, and there were plenty of times I felt discouraged about how I handled a situation. Thankfully, I knew a woman who had parented four kids. She was calm, caring, and always listened to me, and I could call her any time for advice. I learned many of my responses to the girls by watching how she responded to her own children in times of stress. What cemented that learning was being able to talk openly and vulnerably to someone I trusted and respected."

As parents – or simply as people who care about children – we owe it to our children to set a good example. You know: walk the talk, practice what we preach, be the change we want to see in the world. Being a mentor to kids can feel a little like taking a giant pile of inspirational quotes and launching them into action

According to *Mentor: The National Mentoring Partnership*, mentoring "at its core, guarantees young people that there is someone who cares about them, assures them they are not alone in dealing with day-to-day challenges and makes them feel like they matter."

Researchers have found that at-risk kids, particularly those with high absenteeism or behavioral problems, who engaged with a good mentor were far less likely to skip school or use drugs or alcohol and far more likely (55% more) to enroll in college, participate in sports or other extracurricular activities, volunteer regularly or eventually go on to hold leadership positions themselves.

Parents mentor their own children day in and day out, but you may also find you are a mentor to their friends or others outside your normal social circle. Luckily for all of us, being a great mentor – or a great parent – doesn't require perfection. It simply requires commitment to setting a good example and providing the most valuable guidance and support you can to the kids in your life.

## BE THE CHANGE.

What does it take to be a good mentor?

☐ **Be committed:** If you're a parent, it's your job to step up and commit yourself to guiding your own children. If you are not a parent, but choose to mentor another person's child, be 100% certain at the outset that you have the time and emotional bandwidth to help. It could be devastating to start a mentoring relationship only to back out of it before the child is ready.

☐ **Demonstrate character and integrity:** Kids need to know you are a person they can trust. That requires honesty, mature decision making and showing respect for the child – always.

☐ **Be consistent:** Show up for kids when and where you say you will and have a back-up plan for times when plans fall through. Your own kids need to know they can count on you anytime. A child you mentor outside of your family also needs to know that you are true to your word and that you honor your promises. Consistency means doing what you say you will, even when that may involve enforcing negative consequences for a child's behavior.

☐ **Have patience:** Relationships take time. If you mentor someone other than your own child, that child's own past experiences and personality may keep them from opening up or confiding in you right away. Your continued involvement and caring will help break down those barriers.

☐ **Show compassion:** Listen well, but reserve judgment. One of the most difficult aspects of mentoring someone is that they may choose to ignore your advice. That's part of growing up but a hard truth to accept, especially when your own child is the one making poor choices. As a mentor, it's not your job to live somebody else's life, but to continue to support kids even when they experience setbacks. And, you need to recognize that your advice may not always be the best thing for the child.

☐ **Enjoy your time together:** Being a mentor is certainly not all serious business. Play together, laugh together, take turns choosing fun activities and always keep your mind open to learning from the kids you work with. They can be fantastic teachers too.

## AMPLIFY YOUR EFFORTS.

If you feel you have what it takes to formally mentor kids in your community, there is likely a strong need for your services. If one-on-one mentorship feels beyond your current time or commitment availability, you might find opportunities to be part of a less demanding team or group mentorship program. Schools always need volunteers and that could be a great starting point for you. And remember that mentoring in the community may require training to be sure the kids with you are safe. Mentoring should not involve one-on-one isolated time together. You don't ever want your intentions to be questioned.

Do some research to assess the need and opportunities in your local area. You might also check out Big Brothers Big Sisters or www.mentoring.org for connections to programs near you. Value whatever background checking the program conducts to assure that you are appropriate for their activities.

If you have a child who you feel could benefit from having a mentor, contact these same organizations to make a connection.

# RESOURCES:

Ahern K: Five Ways You Can Be a Good Mentor for a Child. NYMetroParents, August 21, 2012. Available at: http://www.nymetroparents.com/article/Five-tips-to-being-a-great-mentor-for-a-child-in-need-20120821.

Connor J: 10 Tips to Mentor Youth Like a Superstar, April 3, 2017. Available at: http://www.drjulieconnor.com/10-mentoring-tips/.

Crutcher BN: Cross Cultural Mentoring Pathway to Making Excellence Inclusive. Association of American Colleges and Universities, Spring 2014, vol 100 (2). Available at: http://www.aacu.org/liberaleducation/2014/spring/crutcher.

Martin J: 7 Steps to Effectively Mentoring Your Kids, 2018. Available at: www.allprodad.com/7-steps-to-effectively-mentoring-your-kids/.

Mentoring.org website. Available at: http://www.mentoring.org/. (Website)

# NOTES:

# 47

# *Support* YOUR SCHOOLS

"When someone says, 'parents are our children's first teachers,' I have to smile because my mother was literally my first teacher. An educator her whole life, she ran the pre-school that I attended. Undoubtedly, her love of learning rubbed off on me as I became a teacher myself. But it was the care she expressed for all my schools – the people, the spaces, the events we shared together – that really sank in. School felt like a safe and healthy place to be, which made me feel like I belonged and everything was going to be okay, even when things were really hard."

15,535. That's how many hours – give or take – kids spend in the classroom from kindergarten until the day they flip their tassel at high school graduation. That breaks down to nearly 2,500 school days spent in the care of teachers – almost seven straight years if you subtract weekends, breaks and holidays. But enough with the math! Let's just put it out there: any place that your child spends that much time should be a place you care about – a lot.

Truth is, family engagement in a child's education is a proven strategy for their success. If we want healthy kids, then it makes sense to advocate for healthy schools. Plus, showing up and pitching in sends a clear message to your kids that learning matters. Research shows that when parents are involved in schools, kids do better – meaning higher grades, less absenteeism, better social skills and improved behavior.

"Involvement" in your child's education can take many forms. Aim to be a partner to the teachers who spend all those hours with your child. At home, reinforce what is being taught at school. Note: DON'T DO your kids' homework for them but be available to provide support as needed. Schools are always in need of volunteers – your time, talent, ideas and energy are appreciated. No matter what you have to offer, there is a place and a need for it.

## SHOW UP, AND LEND YOUR VOICE

Make it your business to get to know your kids' teachers, the principal, the school secretary and anybody else who comes in regular contact with your children. Not sure where to start? We have some ideas for you:

☐ Volunteer in the classroom.

☐ Chaperone a field trip or school dance.

☐ Share your talents: build a set for the school play or lead an art lesson.

☐ Help with fundraising efforts.

☐ Join the PTO (or another parent group).

☐ Attend parent-teacher conferences and back-to-school nights as often as your schedule permits.

☐ Be social! Take the whole family to the school carnival, family night or concerts.

☐ Work shifts at the concession stand during athletic events.

☐ Donate money to help fund extra teachers, special projects or support tight budgets.

☐ **Make connections with other parents at your kids' school.**

☐ **Advocate for school improvements that give kids the resources they need to learn and thrive.**

☐ **See or hear something that doesn't feel right? Speak up!**

At home, make sure your kids know school is a priority. Help them set goals and work toward achieving them. Stay on top of their grades and assignments. Most schools have an online portal for parents to access this information. And, always let them know you're proud of their efforts.

It is understood that not all parents have the same resources, both in terms of money and time, to participate in many school activities, but all parents should try to keep abreast of their child's progress in school and advocate for the services they need. Supporting the work of the school in a larger sense gives all kids, including yours, a boost. Choose a path that offers support, even in a small way, as best you can.

*Parents for Healthy Schools* (see references) has an online quiz you can take to determine the health of your child's school and offers resources to help promote a culture of wellness. It includes questions like:

- Does your school punish students for misbehavior by withholding recess or PE?
- Do classroom/school parties usually feature healthy food and/or physical activity?
- Is your child required to complete a health education course in middle school?
- Does your school have healthy programs for staff and teachers?

It's all food for thought and a place to start in the effort to accelerate positive change in your schools. Your efforts will help your own kids – and everyone else's.

## AMPLIFY YOUR EFFORTS.

School isn't just a place kids go to learn about math, science and reading. It's where they spend a mighty chunk of their formative years, so it's imperative we all advocate for their safety and security.

Never hesitate to ask questions like these:

☐ How does the school ensure that students are never alone 1:1 with an older youth or grown-up?

☐ Is there a code of conduct limiting interactions between staff and children outside of school activities?

☐ Are children receiving any sexual abuse prevention education? If so, are those lessons developmentally appropriate and based on strong evidence of what works?

Important to note: As of February, 2022, 37 states have passed legislation (called Erin's Law) requiring schools to provide child sexual abuse prevention education to K-12 students, staff and families and the law is pending in 12 more states. What is your school doing?

Asking questions and promoting a healthy school environment is a great way to join with other adults, teachers and your own kids to make positive changes that can benefit the whole community.

---

## RESOURCES:

Action for Healthy Kids website. Available at: www. parentsforhealthykids.org.

CDC: Parents for Healthy Schools website, Aug. 8, 2019. Available at: https://www.cdc.gov/healthyschools/parentengagement/ parentsforhealthyschools/p4hs. htm (Also in Spanish)

Erin's Law website. Available at: http://www.erinslaw.org/.

Garcia LE, Thornton O: *The enduring importance of parental involvement*, November 14, 2014. Available at: https://www.neatoday.org/2014/11/18/ the-enduring-importance-of-parental-involvement-2/.

KidsHealth from Nemours: *10 ways to help your child succeed in elementary school*, August, 2018. Available at: www.kidshealth.org/en/parents/school-help-elementary. (Also in Spanish)

Wilder S: Effects of parental involvement on academic achievement. *J. Ed Review* 66:13:377-397, May 14, 2013.

---

# NOTES:

# 48
## VOLUNTEER *Together*

"When I was younger, my parents made a point of finding out what the greatest community needs were in our area, then made sure the whole family took time to help in whatever way we could. Sometimes, we helped elderly neighbors with yard-work, or delivered food to families who were struggling. We regularly volunteered together at a homeless shelter around the holidays. Not only did we come together as a family, we all left feeling like we made a difference for others in our community.

What if you knew that raising your hand more often could help your kids become significantly more compassionate, confident and cooperative humans? Well, you might end up with a repetitive hand-raising stress injury, but we're betting you'd be happy to do it.

This is what volunteering is all about: Raising your hand to help somebody else, actually making a difference in a world where that often feels very, very difficult, and building some character in the process. When you get your children involved and working beside you – what a score for their development! It would be tough to conceive a down side to volunteering, but it may further moti-vate you to know that volunteering:

- Promotes teamwork and cooperation.

- Encourages awareness of what life is like for those less fortunate – reinforcing an appreciation for what we have.
- Builds empathy and sensitivity toward others.
- Introduces new skills, such as leadership, organization and communication.
- Forges connections with others.
- Strengthens bonds with your kids when you volunteer together.
- Makes you happier!

And there's a bonus! Volunteering translates well into the world of college, adulthood, and work. College admissions teams and employers recognize that students who commit to regular volunteer work are often more skilled at time management and likely have some of the very skills and attributes noted above. Volunteering builds character, and everybody wants in on that.

## PUT YOUR INTENTIONS INTO ACTION.

Every community on the planet has needs that can only be met when people come together and pitch in. If you start small and local, you may find it less daunting to figure out the time and logistics.

☐ **Choose a cause that resonates with both you and your children**. Volunteer opportunities that work for even preschool age kids include: visiting a nursing/retirement home, adopting a family for the holidays, assisting at an animal shelter, pitching in at park or community cleanup projects, or delivering meals to the elderly or disabled.

☐ **Don't stress about the time commitment**. Do what feels right and works for you. By simply choosing to make volunteering a regular part of your family life, you send a powerful message to your kids and can help set them up for a life of service to others. What a beautiful thing!

☐ **Encourage your children to participate in school, church, or community-sponsored volunteer activities**. Perhaps there is a fun-run to collect money for a good cause. Organizations like *Special Olympics* often need young helpers to assist children with developmental challenges. Scouting organizations are also typically focused on supporting kids in doing good in their community. Sometimes there are opportunities to work with a group to improve the property of a person who doesn't have the resources to make needed changes.

## AMPLIFY YOUR EFFORTS.

If you manage to spark a fire of philanthropy in your child, well done! You could end up with a super-motivated young person who wants to light up the world. Help them.

Taking volunteering to the next level could mean helping your child:

- Organize a school food, clothing or money collection to benefit a favorite charity or community need.
- Work to motivate other kids to volunteer as a group for different causes.
- Start their very own non-profit.

Whatever they choose, be their champion and partner. The world needs their – and *your* – service.

---

# RESOURCES:

Children's Bureau: *10 benefits of volunteering at a non-profit*. Available at: http://www.all4kids. org/2017/09/28/10-benefits-of-volunteering-at-a-non-profit/.

Families for Life: *7 reasons why your child should volunteer*, 2019. Available at: http://www.familiesforlife.sg/discover-an-article/ Pages/7-Reasons-Why-Your-Child-Should-Volunteer.aspx.

International School of Minnesota: *Eight great was kids benefit from volunteer work*, 2017. Available at: https://www.internationalschoolmn.com/news-blog/blog/eight-great-ways-kids-benefit-from-volunteer-work.

Onion A: *How to volunteer with kids*, 2016. Available at: http://www.sittercity.com/parents/family-activities/how-to-volunteer-with-kids.

---

# NOTES:

# 49

## CULTIVATE AN ATTITUDE OF GRATITUDE

"As a child, my mom prompted me to think about what I was grateful for every day, whether at dinner table conversations or in my bed time prayers. Today, as the mother of a two-year-old, I look for ways to infuse a grateful attitude into our daily lives – a verbal 'thank you' to the daycare workers at the end of a long day, thanking my husband for a homemade dinner, telling my son how happy I am that he's helping pick up his toys before bedtime. As my son gets older, I look forward to deeper conversations and community service opportunities that will help to remind us of how much we truly have to be thankful for."

Gratitude, it has been said, is one of the greatest virtues. Throughout history, gratitude has also been characterized as an emotion, a skill, an attitude, and a "social glue." In recent years, studying gratitude has become a science: as it turns out, a sense of gratitude is embedded in our very DNA.

So why do some people seem naturally better at expressing gratitude than others? The reasons are likely endless, but fortunately for all of us and our kids, there are ways we can practice boosting our sense of gratitude to bring more fullness to our lives.

According to experts, adopting an "attitude of gratitude" has tremendous benefits. As outlined by gratitude expert Dr. Robert

A. Emmons of the University of California, Davis, these include better sleep, increased self-esteem, hope, empathy, and optimism, as well as more positive perceptions of school and family. Dr. Emmons suggests that grateful people are *happier* people—by as much as 25%!

Gratitude is also a critical building block for healthy relationships. Identifying what we're grateful for heightens our awareness of the people and things that make our lives worthwhile. And that kind of appreciation leads to more respectful behavior.

## SERVE UP SOME APPRECIATION.

Given the boost we derive from gratitude, it's important to get kids off on the right foot. Developing a grateful disposition takes time, effort and practice, starting early in childhood.

Here are four ways to get and *keep* the ball rolling:

☐ **Model gratitude.** Make a point of expressing your appreciation for all sorts of things out loud—sincerely and often. And remember—kids can tell when you're faking it.

☐ **Don't overload the house with "things."** Buying everything your kids ask for doesn't guarantee their happiness And it may drive you bankrupt. Help your children understand the difference between *wants* and *needs*—and ensure their appreciation of both by keeping purchases modest. By talking with children about the cost of things like toys, you'll also be contributing to their financial education which is often overlooked both at home and in school.

☐ **Instill a work ethic and the value of giving back.** It's not unreasonable to ask kids to help around the house, even at an early age. In fact, two-and-three-year-olds are great at turning tasks such as setting the table into a game. Not only does their success at age-appropriate chores build self-esteem, it helps them appreciate everything else that goes into running a home—and caring for others. You might incentivize more difficult and time-consuming jobs with a modest allowance.

Cultivating gratitude—like all virtues—is a process. The more you stick with it, the better the results. And while there are bound to be some rough edges—especially around chores—*someday* (and we're probably talking years here) your kids might even thank *you* for the effort.

## AMPLIFY YOUR EFFORTS.

☐ **Start a new tradition.** When you sit down for a meal or tuck your kids into bed, ask them to share what they're grateful for *today* and share what you're grateful for as well. Another nice exercise is writing thank you notes together. Even one-year-olds enjoy scribbling—which makes for original cards that are cherished by recipients!

☐ **Find an age-appropriate community service opportunity to do together – even if it's baking cookies for a neighbor who needs cheering up.** These types of experiences tend to take all of us out of our own internal lives, waking us up to the needs and struggles of others. Most young kids are naturally attuned to those in need. Helping them respond appropriately is another way to extend their appreciation for what they already have. Choosing toys or books they no longer use to give to a charity for other children is another way to help them learn to share graciously.

☐ **Keep reminding your kids what matters most.** People come from different backgrounds, income levels, and educational histories. But no matter what we have or lack in the way of material things, it's the people we choose to surround ourselves with that leads to lasting pleasure and helps build the supportive community we all need to lift us up.

# RESOURCES:

Bergstrom C: *Mindfulness exercise for children: gratitude for happiness and health*, 2015. Available at: www.blissfulkids.com/mindfulness-exercises-for-children-gratitude-happiness-and-health/.

Froh J, Bono G: *Seven ways to foster gratitude in kids.* Available at: http://www.greatergood.berkeley.edu/article/item/seven_ways_to_foster_gratitude_in_kids.

Reiser A: *11 tips for instilling true gratitude in your kids*, 2014. Available at: http://www.huffingtonpost.com/andrea-reiser/11-tips-for-instilling-true-gratitude-in-your-kids_b_4708019.html.

Allen, Summer Ph.D.: *The Science of Gratitude.* Available at:https://ggsc.berkeley.edu/images/uploads/GGSC-JTF_White_Paper-Gratitude-FINAL.pdf

# NOTES:

# 50
## BE *Resilient*

"Sometimes when I'm trying to teach my son about resilience, I realize the lesson might be just as much (or more!) for me than him. And I have that 'aha moment' of thinking that we should both be taking deep breaths, turning off screens, moving our bodies, exploring new creative solutions to problems, and naming our feelings without giving them more power than they should have. Then other times I tell him, 'Mom needs a timeout,' and go up to my bedroom to watch a reality show and drink a glass of wine. And to me, this balance is all about what resilience is – sometimes it's built by a new way of thinking about things, and sometimes your resilience increases just by taking a much-needed break."

Here's the thing about parenting. (Let's be real. There are *many* "things" about parenting, but this is a big one.) Before you had kids, you were in charge of *you*. That's it – and some days, even that felt like one too many people to worry about. When life got hard, or emotional, or skidded sideways, you could temporarily just check out.

Then, along came another human and checking out was no longer an option. Yet, the same challenges, plus a whole pile of new ones, remained.

Becoming a parent doesn't magically erase the trauma or

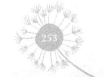

stressors you may have experienced. Far from it. Life throws curve balls. We catch some, dodge others, and once in a while get bonked – hard enough to knock the wind out of us. It can feel overwhelming.

How we handle those setbacks says a ton about our *resilience:* our ability to take a hit, get back up, and stay in the game. If you've got it, life is undoubtedly easier to navigate.

For adults who experienced childhood trauma such as abuse or neglect, parenthood may trigger deep emotions – especially if their child faces similar circumstances. Other life stressors – including health, marital, financial, or domestic violence issues – can also impact a parent's ability to fully support their children day in and day out.

The fantastic news is that resilience is partially innate but it can be learned, built, and strengthened. It's never too late to start. As airline flight attendants like to tell us: put on your own oxygen mask before helping your children. When you're equipped to tackle what life throws at you, you're in a much better position to help your children do the same.

## BOUNCING BACK

Boost your resilience by adopting some new ways of thinking. Easier said than done—but definitely worth the effort. Try these out:

- Remind yourself – often – that most problems are surmountable.
- At the same time, accept that some things can't be changed.

So, change what you can, recognize what you can't, and move on.

But what about your kids and resilience? Resilience is the ability to bounce back from adversity, stress, failure, disappointment. And much as you want to protect them, your kids will face some bad times in their young lives. Moving, divorce, death of a family member or pet, abuse, bullying, or illness are all things that kids may face and, to them, they are huge problems. Once kids learn that they can overcome difficulties, they will also learn that they are strong and capable people. Figuring it all out takes time, but you can help. A few strategies to try:

☐ **Build emotional connections with them so that they feel your support.**

☐ **Promote healthy risk-taking.** This gives kids the practice they need to move outside their comfort zone but without involving huge risks. Some kids are natural adventurers while others are more anxious about leaping to try a new sport or activity, talk with someone new, or even sample a new food. Encourage them to push past their fears.

☐ **Resist the urge to fix your child's problems.** Certainly, you should be there for support and advice, but try not to take over the situation. Instead, engage your child in problem-solving. Ask them: What can you try? What might happen? Where could you get some help?

☐ **Help your child to label his or her feelings.** Understand that fear or anxiety are signs of stress and that relief is also a feeling to be aware of.

☐ **Demonstrate coping skills such as deep breathing before starting a new activity.**

☐ **Help your child to be optimistic in the face of adversity.** Ask them: What good might come out of this experience?

☐ **Embrace the learning that comes from making mistakes.** Outcomes don't need to be perfect, but there is almost always something positive that can be learned from a challenging event or situation.

## AMPLIFY YOUR EFFORTS.

When your child is successful in coping with a stressful situation, remind them of their success when the next stressor comes along. Build their resilience one situation at a time.

☐ Be mindful that some situations may be too stressful for

a child to work through, even with parental help. *If severe trauma has been experienced, seek professional support.* Call your primary care provider, Child Advocacy Center, school counselor, or other professional source for help for yourself and your family. And reinforce that knowing when to seek help is also a critical lesson in resilience.

# RESOURCES:

American Psychological Association (APA): *The road to resilience*, 2019. Available at: http://www.apa.org/helpcenter/road-resilience.

Brandt A: *9 steps to healing childhood trauma as an adult*, 2018. Available at: http://www.psychologytoday.com/us/blog/mindful-anger/201804/9-steps-healing-childhood-trauma-adult

Daskal L: *How to be more resilient when things get tough*, 2015. Available at: https://www.inc.com/lolly-daskal/how-to-be-more-resilient-when-things-get-tough.html

Hurley K: *Resilience in children: Strategies to strengthen your kids*. Available at: www.psycom.net/build-resilience-children

National Foundation to End Child Abuse: *How do you teach children resilience*. ENDCAN. Available at: https://endcan.org/2020/05/19/how-do-you-teach-children-resilience

Tartakovsky Tartakovsky M: *10 tips for raising resilient kids*, 2018. Available at: https://psychcentral.com/lib/10-tips-for-raising-resilient-kids#1.

U. S. Department of Health and Human Services, Children's Bureau, Child Welfare Information Gateway: *Parental resilience resources*, no date. Available at: www.childwelfare.gov/topics/preventing/promoting/protectfactors/resilience/.

Resilitator.com: *Resiliency: Nature or Nurture?*, 2015. Available at: www.resilitator.com/index.php/resiliency-reader/38-resiliency-nautre-or-nurture

Suttie J: *Four ways social support makes you more resilient*, November 13, 2017. Available at: https://www.greatergood.berkeley.edu/article/item/four_ways_social_support_makes_you_more_resilient

---

# NOTES:

# ACKNOWLEDGMENTS

Our goal – and hope – is that this book will inspire parents and others who care for children to build a better, safer world for them. We want families to enjoy raising their children, and to take pride in knowing that they are doing the best they can to raise them happy, healthy, safe, and listened to.

Many people have helped us to bring this book to publication. We want to thank the Children's Center Staff & Board for their work in bringing forward ideas about how to prevent child abuse through building stronger families and communities. A special thanks to Karen Rush, PhD, Executive Director, for her outstanding editing assistance and leadership to bring the book across the finish line.

John & June Rogers believe in child abuse prevention and contributed funds to help underwrite the project.

Many people reviewed the book to assure that a balanced Diversity, Equity, and Inclusion framework was maintained.

Ardys Dunn, PhD, PNP-r; Catherine Blosser, MPH, PNP-r; Pam Avila, FNP; and others all contributed to the book's completion. We are appreciative of the suggestions and work of each of them.

Masha Shubin helped us take the manuscript to a published book format.

Thank you to all!

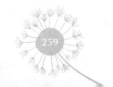

# ABOUT THE AUTHOR, EDITOR, AND CHILDREN'S CENTER

## KAREN LUNDERGAN FRIESEN, B.S.

*Karen has a Bachelor's degree in Journalism from the University of Portland. She is the parent of three children, and has experience as a Court Appointed Special Advocate (CASA) working with abused children.*

## CATHERINE BURNS, PHD, FAAN - EDITOR

*Catherine is a retired Pediatric and Family Nurse Practitioner Educator and Professor emeritus, Oregon Health Sciences University School of Nursing, Portland, OR. She was the lead author of eight textbooks related to pediatric primary care and is a retired Children's Center Board Member. She is the mother of two and the grandmother of four.*

## ABOUT THE CHILDREN'S CENTER
## OREGON CITY, OREGON

**The Children's Center** *is a Child Advocacy Center where children and families experiencing abuse, neglect, or domestic violence can receive assessments and intervention support. Child Advocacy Centers also work to prevent abuse through community-oriented activities. The authors encourage readers to learn more about their local Child Abuse Advocacy Center by visiting the National Child Advocacy Center at* www.nationalcac.org.

*All proceeds from sales of this book will benefit the Children's Center.*

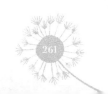

261

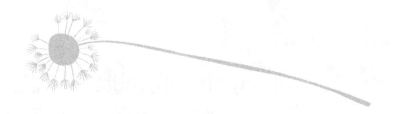

# CHILDHELP

## *National Child Abuse Hotline*

**If You Suspect Child Abuse Or Neglect, Call This Number
To Reach Your State's Child Abuse Help Services:**

# 1-800-422-4453

Your call will be confidential

## (www.childhelp.org/hotline)

# PLEASE WRITE A BOOK REVIEW FOR US

What did you think of *Raising Happy, Healthy, Safe kids: 50 Tips for Tackling Even the Toughest Challenges with Love, Joy, and Purpose?*

If you enjoyed this book and found it beneficial, we invite you to post a review on www.Amazon/books or whatever website you used to purchase it.

Thank you!

CPSIA information can be obtained
at www.ICGtesting.com
Printed in the USA
BVHW051525240423
662929BV00005B/6